OTHER FAST FACTS BOOKS

Fast Facts on **ADOLESCENT HEALTH FOR NURSING AND HEALTH PROFESSIONALS**: A Care Guide (*Herrman*)

Fast Facts for the **ADULT-GERONTOLOGY ACUTE CARE NURSE PRACTITIONER** (*Carpenter*)

Fast Facts for the **ANTEPARTUM AND POSTPARTUM NURSE**: A Nursing Orientation and Care Guide (*Davidson*)

Fast Facts Workbook for **CARDIAC DYSRHYTHMIAS AND 12-LEAD EKGs** (*Desmarais*)

Fast Facts for the **CARDIAC SURGERY NURSE**: Caring for Cardiac Surgery Patients, Third Edition (*Hodge*)

Fast Facts for **CAREER SUCCESS IN NURSING**: Making the Most of Mentoring (*Vance*)

Fast Facts for the **CATH LAB NURSE,** Second Edition (*McCulloch*)

Fast Facts for the **CLASSROOM NURSING INSTRUCTOR**: Classroom Teaching (*Yoder-Wise, Kowalski*)

Fast Facts for the **CLINICAL NURSE LEADER** (*Wilcox, Deerhake*)

Fast Facts for the **CLINICAL NURSE MANAGER**: Managing a Changing Workplace, Second Edition (*Fry*)

Fast Facts for the **CLINICAL NURSING INSTRUCTOR**: Clinical Teaching, Third Edition (*Kan, Stabler-Haas*)

Fast Facts on **COMBATING NURSE BULLYING, INCIVILITY, AND WORKPLACE VIOLENCE**: What Nurses Need to Know (*Ciocco*)

Fast Facts About **COMPETENCY-BASED EDUCATION IN NURSING**: How to Teach Competency Mastery (*Wittmann-Price, Gittings*)

Fast Facts for the **CRITICAL CARE NURSE,** Second Edition (*Hewett*)

Fast Facts About **CURRICULUM DEVELOPMENT IN NURSING**: How to Develop and Evaluate Educational Programs, Second Edition (*McCoy, Anema*)

Fast Facts for **DEMENTIA CARE**: What Nurses Need to Know, Second Edition (*Miller*)

Fast Facts for **DEVELOPING A NURSING ACADEMIC PORTFOLIO**: What You Really Need to Know (*Wittmann-Price*)

Fast Facts for **DNP ROLE DEVELOPMENT**: A Career Navigation Guide (*Menonna-Quinn, Tortorella Genova*)

Fast Facts About **EKGs FOR NURSES**: The Rules of Identifying EKGs (*Landrum*)

Fast Facts for the **ER NURSE**: Guide to a Successful Emergency Department Orientation, Fourth Edition (*Buettner*)

Fast Facts for **EVIDENCE-BASED PRACTICE IN NURSING**: Third Edition (*Godshall*)

Fast Facts for the **FAITH COMMUNITY NURSE**: Implementing FCN/Parish Nursing (*Hickman*)

Fast Facts About **FORENSIC NURSING**: What You Need to Know (*Scannell*)

Fast Facts for the **GERONTOLOGY NURSE**: A Nursing Care Guide (*Eliopoulos*)

Fast Facts About **GI AND LIVER DISEASES FOR NURSES**: What APRNs Need to Know (*Chaney*)

FAST FACTS for
THE L&D NURSE

Kathryn "Cassie" Giles Groll, DNP, CNM, IBCLC, is a doctorally prepared, certified nurse midwife who is part of a full-scope OB/GYN private practice in New Jersey. She earned her master's degree in nursing and doctoral degree from the University of Medicine and Dentistry of New Jersey. She is licensed in both New Jersey and New York as a certified nurse midwife with prescriptive authority and as an OB/GYN nurse practitioner in the state of New York. Dr. Groll has worked as a midwife since 2006 and clinically as an RN in obstetrics in a variety of capacities, including as a clinical instructor of obstetrics at Columbia University, New York, and in the high-risk women's health float pool at NewYork-Presbyterian/Weill Cornell Medical Center, New York. She is a member of the American College of Nurse-Midwives, the Medical History Society of New Jersey, and Sigma Theta Tau International Honor Society of Nursing. She has served as an advocate for sexual assault victims in Somerset, New Jersey.

FAST FACTS for
THE L&D NURSE

Labor and Delivery Orientation

Third Edition

Cassie Giles Groll, DNP, CNM, IBCLC

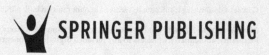

First Springer Publishing edition 2012; subsequent edition 2015.

Springer Publishing Company, LLC
11 West 42nd Street, New York, NY 10036
www.springerpub.com
connect.springerpub.com/

Acquisitions Editor: Rachel Landes
Compositor: Transforma

ISBN: 978-0-8261-5124-7
ebook ISBN: 978-0-8261-5131-5
DOI: 10.1891/9780826151315

Printed by BnT

The author and the publisher of this Work have made every effort to use sources believed to be reliable to provide information that is accurate and compatible with the standards generally accepted at the time of publication. Because medical science is continually advancing, our knowledge base continues to expand. Therefore, as new information becomes available, changes in procedures become necessary. We recommend that the reader always consult current research and specific institutional policies before performing any clinical procedure or delivering any medication. The author and publisher shall not be liable for any special, consequential, or exemplary damages resulting, in whole or in part, from the readers' use of, or reliance on, the information contained in this book. The publisher has no responsibility for the persistence or accuracy of URLs for external or third-party Internet websites referred to in this publication and does not guarantee that any content on such websites is, or will remain, accurate or appropriate.

Library of Congress Cataloging-in-Publication Data
Names: Groll, Cassie Giles, author.
Title: Fast facts for the L&D nurse: labor and delivery orientation /
  Kathryn "Cassie" Giles Groll.
Other titles: Fast facts for the labor and delivery nurse | Fast facts
  (Springer Publishing Company)
Description: Third edition. | New York, NY : Springer Publishing Company, [2022] | Series: Fast
  facts | Includes bibliographical references and index. | Summary: "The third edition of this book
  continues to provide basic information pertaining to standard obstetric practices commonly seen
  in labor and delivery (L&D). Its intent is to allow the senior staff to focus on more emergent questions new nurses may have rather than the basics of their environment. This edition provides the
  direction needed for new nurses to develop a comfortable independence and confidence in the
  labor and delivery environment"– Provided by publisher.
Identifiers: LCCN 2021970070 | ISBN 9780826151247 (paperback) | ISBN
  9780826151315 (ebook)
Subjects: MESH: Delivery, Obstetric–nursing | Obstetric Nursing–methods |
  Labor, Obstetric. | Obstetric Labor Complications–nursing
Classification: LCC RG951 | NLM WY 157 | DDC 618.2/0231–dc23/eng/20220106
LC record available at https://lccn.loc.gov/2021970070

Contact sales@springerpub.com to receive discount rates on bulk purchases.

Printed in the United States of America.

This book is dedicated to my children, Cooper and Charlotte. You have both brought me so much happiness and laughter. I cannot imagine my world without you. I live and breathe every second for our next hug. I am so proud of you and the little people you have become. And to my husband, Chris, without whose undying support and immense patience, nothing would be possible. I love you! Also to my parents, who have supported me so that I could have everything I have today.

Contents

Part I GENERAL ORIENTATION AND LABOR AND DELIVERY OVERVIEW

Part II PROCEDURES

Part III EMERGENCIES

Preface

The third edition of this book continues to provide basic information pertaining to standard obstetric practices commonly seen in labor and delivery (L&D). Its intent is to allow senior staff to focus on more emergent questions new nurses may have rather than the basics of their environment. This edition provides the direction needed for new nurses to develop a comfortable independence and confidence in the L&D environment.

As with the first and second editions, the purpose of this book is not to overwhelm the nurse with information but to provide a tool that is simple in use and format. It provides clear instructions on what to do, equipment needed, and whom to call in the event of an emergency. It does not take the place of practitioner orders or institutional guidelines.

As the face of medicine changes, the need to use the term *provider* instead of *physician* or *doctor* is indicated. Certified nurse midwives are gaining more and more popularity in the obstetric community, including in private midwifery practices and private physicians' offices. There is much misunderstanding of what exactly a certified nurse midwife does and what the scope of practice is. A certified nurse midwife is a highly skilled, uniquely trained nurse in the field of normal obstetrics and gynecology. They can order drugs, deliver babies, and do in-office and L&D procedures, as well as assist in surgery. In many hospitals, midwives help train residents. Most midwives who deliver out of hospitals believe in pain medications for their patients and are highly skilled in emergency situations. They have achieved a postgraduate education, and many of them hold doctoral degrees in the field of nursing or other health-related fields. The regulations and scope of practice vary from state to state, and if you have any questions about what midwives can do on your unit, be sure to ask senior nursing staff or consult your institutional protocols.

Fast Facts for the L&D Nurse, Third Edition, has been completely updated to reflect the newest evidence-based practice guidelines from the American College of Obstetricians and Gynecologists and the Society of Maternal-Fetal Medicine. Chapters cover the more commonly occurring L&D situations and introduce unfamiliar terminology, equipment, labs, medications, and algorithms. Important topics in each section are alphabetized for ease of reference, and many clear illustrations aid learning. New illustrations are introduced that depict and facilitate understanding of effacement and dilatation of the cervix, breech presentation and delivery, umbilical cord prolapse, placental abruption, and others, and additional clinical practice information is highlighted in "Fast Facts" boxes. There are also two new and useful appendices: a quick-reference appendix for most commonly referenced clinical charts and tables and an additional new appendix containing an alphabetically ordered synopsis of important drug-related information with L&D and nursing implications.

A special note to the nurses who use this guide: It is a great responsibility to be an L&D nurse. Although there are days you will forget and will see that day as just another day at work, remember it is one of the most amazing days in the life of your patient and that she should be met and guided through this process with the same enthusiasm you would want to surround the birth of your own child. It is also important to remember that as a new life enters this world, they should be greeted with love and joyfulness, with profound happiness that they are here. You should always be humbled by the fact that it is a privilege to be part of a miracle.

Acknowledgments

I want to express my deepest gratitude to Dr. Elaine Diegmann, CNM, ND, and Dr. Labib Riachi, MD. Elaine, thank you for believing in me and teaching me how to be a midwife. You have given me the most amazing gift: the ability to partake in a miracle. I am extraordinarily lucky to have been your student. Special thanks to my friend and mentor, Dr. Riachi, who through the years has been more than generous with his time and expertise.

This book would not have been possible without my expert panel: Dr. Elaine Diegmann, CNM, ND; Dr. Ginette Lange, CNM, PhD; Dr. Joyce Hyatt, CNM, DNP; and Ruth Monchek, CNM. Your input and immense knowledge were invaluable to this process.

To my friend, Dr. Rachel Behrendt, DNP, I thank you for graciously offering your expertise in proofreading.

And finally, thanks to my husband, Chris, for volunteering to help with the medical illustrations. Your talent is beyond words and has made this book visually beautiful. Thank you!

Contributor, Part III

Terri Thompson, DNP, RN
Associate Professor of Nursing
College of Nursing
California Baptist University

I

GENERAL ORIENTATION AND LABOR AND DELIVERY OVERVIEW

This section presents common occurrences during labor and delivery (L&D). It covers definitions, everyday terminology, and common actions with which you should become totally familiar. The section presents a review of medications you may come in contact with on a daily basis, including their indications and common dosages. Remember, in the L&D unit, you have two patients and your actions must take both patients into account.

Medications to Know—generic (trade)

- Betamethasone (Celestone)
- Butorphanol (Stadol)
- Calcium gluconate
- Carboprost (Hemabate)
- Citric acid/sodium citrate (Bicitra)
- Dexamethasone
- Dinoprostone (Cervidil)
- Ephedrine
- Erythromycin ophthalmic ointment
- Hydralazine
- Indomethacin (Indocin)
- Insulin
- Labetalol (Trandate)
- Lidocaine (Xylocaine)
- Magnesium sulfate
- Meperidine (Demerol)
- Methylergonovine (Methergine)
- Misoprostol (Cytotec)
- Morphine
- Nalbuphine (Nubain)
- Naloxone
- Nifedipine (Procardia)
- Oxytocin (Pitocin)
- Promethazine (Phenergan)
- Rho(D) immunoglobulin, human (IGIM) (RhoGAM)
- Terbutaline
- Vitamin K (phytonadione)

Abbreviations to Learn

- AFI—amniotic fluid index
- AFP—alpha fetoprotein
- AROM—artificial rupture of membranes
- CVS—chorionic villa sampling
- DKA—diabetic ketoacidosis
- EDC—estimated date of confinement
- EFW—estimated fetal weight
- FHR—fetal heart rate
- GBS—group B *Streptococcus*
- GC/CT—gonorrhea/*Chlamydia trachomatis*
- GDM—gestational diabetes mellitus

- HBsAg—hepatitis B surface antigen
- ISE—internal scalp electrode
- IUPC—intrauterine pressure catheter
- IUFD—intrauterine fetal demise
- LGA/SGA—large for gestational age/small for gestational age
- LMP—last menstrual period
- MVU—Montevideo units
- NSVD—normal spontaneous vaginal delivery
- PPROM—preterm premature rupture of membranes
- ROM—rupture of membranes
- SROM—spontaneous rupture of membranes
- Toco—tocodynamometer
- UCX—uterine contractions
- U/S—ultrasound
- VBAC—vaginal birth after cesarean section

Equipment to Locate and Become Familiar With
- Allis clamps
- Blades
- Bovie tip
- Compression boots
- Curved Kellys
- Electrosurgery hookup
- Forceps
- Infant pulse oximeter
- Infant warmer
- Infusion pump
- Kochers
- Lap sponges
- Needle holders
- Nitrazine paper
- Pulse oximeter
- Ring forceps
- Scalpels
- Scissors
- Self-retaining retractors
- Speculum
- Straight Halsteds
- Suction hookup
- Suction tips
- Surgical instruments

- T-clamps
- Tenaculum
- Towel clips
- Tube occluding forceps
- Umbilical cord clamp

AMNIOTIC FLUID

Composed mostly of fetal urine; the volume differs depending on gestational age. It protects and cushions the fetus and contributes to GI tract and lung maturity and development.

Amniotic Fluid Index (AFI)

- U/S is used to measure AFI.
- Abdomen is divided into four quadrants, and the largest pocket of fluid in each quadrant is measured.
- At least one pocket of fluid needs to be 2 × 2 cm or greater or have an AFI total greater than 5.
- No cord or fetal parts should be present in the pocket.
- A normal index is greater than 5 cm and less than 24 cm at term.

Oligohydramnios—AFI Less Than 5 cm at Term

Causes
- Rupture of membranes (ROM)
- Genitourinary malformation
- Postdates
- Placental insufficiency

Risks
- Prolonged ROM may lead to infection
- Continued oligohydramnios may cause malformation
- Cord compression leading to fetal hypoxia (nonreassuring tracing), you will often see variables and amnioinfusion may be ordered
- Fetal demise

Interventions
- IV fluids for mother
- Antibiotics if preterm
- Induction of labor if term

If patient is in labor, continuous fetal monitoring is possible by amnioinfusion.

Polyhydramnios—AFI Greater Than 24 cm at Term

Causes
- Diabetes mellitus
- Maternal substance abuse
- Tracheoesophageal malformation
- Neural tube defects
- Chromosomal abnormalities
- Twin-to-twin transfusion syndrome

Risks
- Unstable lie of fetus
- Cord prolapse with SROM or AROM

Interventions
- In labor
  - Controlled AROM (needle point) to prevent SROM
  - U/S for fetal lie if patient is in labor
- If preterm
  - Amnioreduction
  - Indomethacin (Indocin) 25 mg PO q 6 hr × 48 hr to reduce fetal urine production

Assessment of Rupture of Membranes (ROM)

Visual
- Sterile speculum inserted into vagina
  - Pooling of fluid noted at fornix of cervix or in vaginal vault
- If unsure, patient should cough to visualize escape of fluid from cervix

Ferning
- Sterile speculum inserted into vagina
  - Use cotton swab to obtain fluid
  - Smear on slide
- If positive ROM, ferning pattern will be seen under microscope

pH Balance Assessment
- Sterile speculum inserted into vagina
  - Touch nitrazine paper to noted fluid
  - Normal vaginal pH when pregnant is less than 4.5
  - Amniotic fluid pH is less than 7.0
- Nitrazine paper/swab changes color to blue at pH less than 7.0

Note: Some vaginal infections can cause vaginal pH to reach levels of 7.0 or greater.

Amniotic Fluid Protein
- Obtain before vaginal exam
  - No speculum necessary
  - Insert swab into vagina
  - If placental alpha microglobulin-1 is present, test will be positive for ROM
- Follow directions for specific product used by individual institution

Sources

Cunningham, G., & Leveno, K. J. (2018). *Williams obstetrics* (25th ed.). McGraw-Hill.

King, T., Brucker, M., Osborne, K., & Jevitt, C. M. (2018). *Varney's midwifery* (6th ed.). Jones & Bartlett Learning.

Simpson, K. R., & Creehan, P. A. (2021). *AWHONN perinatal nursing* (5th ed.). Wolters Kluwer Health.

ANTEPARTUM TESTS

Initial Visit 8 to 12 Weeks
- U/S for dating
- Pap
- Blood type/Rh factor
- Antibody screen
- GC/CT
- Complete blood count (CBC)
- Syphilis
- HIV
- Hepatitis B
- Rubella titer
- UA
- Hemoglobin electrophoresis
- Cystic fibrosis
- Varicella titers
- Toxoplasmosis
- Cytomegalovirus (CMV)
- Blood glucose (if overweight or history of GDM)

U/S, ultrasound; UA, urinanalysis, GC/CT, gonorrhea/*Chlamydia trachomatis*; GDM, gestational diabetes mellitus

11 to 13 Weeks NIPT
- First-trimester screening (blood work and U/S) for early detection of Down syndrome
  - CVS if needed

15 to 18 Weeks
- AFP for early detection of neural tube defects
- QUAD if no first trimester screening done or if increased risk for Down syndrome
- Amniocentesis if needed (most commonly done between 16 and 22 weeks)
- Glucose screening if patient has high-risk factors, including obesity, Hx of GDM, family hx

20 Weeks
- U/S for fetal anatomy

28 Weeks
- If patient is Rh negative, RhoGAM should be administered. (Repeat blood type and Rh factor before administration.)

- CBC
- HIV in some states or in high-risk women
- Glucose test

34 to 36 Weeks

- GBS (test accurate only for 5 weeks if done at 34 weeks and delivering at 41 weeks; consult with the provider if they want to repeat test)
- GC/CT
- Syphilis
- NST/BPP for advanced maternal age, obesity, GDMA, HTN, and other maternal factors such as drug abuse

Sources

Chou, B., Bienstock, J. L., & Satin, A. J. (2021). *The Johns Hopkins manual of gynecology and obstetrics* (6th ed.). Wolters Kluwer Health.

King, T., Brucker, M., Osborne, K., & Jevitt, C. M. (2018). *Varney's midwifery* (6th ed.). Jones & Bartlett Learning.

APGAR SCORE

- A score between 0 and 2 measuring heart rate, muscle tone, respiration rate, color, and reflex of the neonate at 1, 5, and 10 minutes of life

Breathing		
0	1	2
Not breathing	Slow irregular	Crying
Heart Rate		
0	1	2
No heartbeat	Less than 100	Greater than 100
Muscle Tone		
0	1	2
Floppy	Some tone	Active movement
Reflex/Grimace		
0	1	2
No response	Facial grimace only	Pulls away, cries, coughs, or sneezes
Skin color		
0	1	2
Pale blue	Body pink, hands and feet blue	Entire body is pink

Scoring the Apgar

- 1 minute
  - Apgar scores are not indicative of future fetal well-being
- 5 minutes
  - 0 to 3 may indicate future neurological problems
  - 4 to 6 intermediate scores
  - 7 to 10 considered normal scoring range
- 10 minutes
  - Should continue to be assessed every 5 minutes if Apgar remains less than 7

Pediatrician should be called in for delivery for

- Operative delivery
- Maternal infection or fever
- Nonreassuring fetal tracing

Fast Fact

Notify the pediatrician immediately if Apgar score is less than 7 at any time.

Sources

KidsHealth. (2011). *What is the Apgar score?* http://kidshealth.org/parent/ pregnancy_center/q_a/apgar.html#cat32

Simpson, K. R., & Creehan, P. A. (2021). *AWHONN perinatal nursing* (5th ed.). Wolters Kluwer Health.

AROMATHERAPY

Aromatherapy has become very popular for anxiety and pain relief. Many evidence-based studies show positive effects for women in labor. Essential oils can be used through a diffuser or topically in a carrier oil. Mixing two or more essential oils together can heighten the desired effect. Always ask before you use oil and test the mother's sensitivity before using in her labor room.

Anxiety and Stress
- Lavender
- Clary sage
- Jasmine
- Chamomile
- Marjoram

Energy
- Lemon
- Peppermint (also helps with nausea)
- Sweet orange
- Spearmint
- Rosemary
- Ginger (also helps with nausea)

Fast Fact

Eucalyptus globulus is not recommended for children younger than 2 and should not be used in the delivery room.

Source

Ghiasi, A., Bagheri, L., & Haseli, A. (2019). A systematic review on the anxiolytic effect of aromatherapy during the first stage of labor. *Journal of Caring Sciences*, 8(1), 51–60. https://doi.org/10.15171/jcs.2019.008

BISHOP SCORE

Scoring system used to determine whether the cervix is inducible or which induction method would be most successful for a vaginal delivery.

Cervix	Bishop Score			
	0	1	2	3
Dilation	0 cm	1–2 cm	3–4	>5 cm
Effacement	0%–30%	40%–50%	60%–70%	80%
Station	−3	−2	−1/0	+1/+2
Consistency	Firm	Medium	Soft	
Position	Posterior	Mild	Anterior	

From your final total of the Bishop score:

- Add 1 for each previous vaginal delivery and/or if patient is preeclamptic
- Subtract 1 for no prior vaginal deliveries if postdates or PPROM
  - Greater than 4 is considered to be favorable for induction.
  - Less than 4 would need cervical ripening agent or delaying induction if possible.

Sources

American College of Obstetricians and Gynecologists. (2009). ACOG Practice Bulletin No. 107: Induction of labor. *Obstetrics & Gynecology, 114* (Issue 2, Pt.1), 386–397. https://doi.org/10.1097/AOG.0b013e3181b48ef5

Cunningham, G., & Leveno, K. J. (2018). *Williams obstetrics* (25th ed.). McGraw-Hill.

BREASTFEEDING

Breastfeeding should be initiated immediately after delivery or as soon as possible. Encourage skin-to-skin contact throughout the couple's hospital stay to maximize the opportunity for exclusive breastfeeding. The infant should be offered the breast, not forced, as this has shown to make latching more difficult or painful. When infant is properly latched you should hear a *Kha-Kha-Kha* sound, which is the sound of the baby swallowing.

If you hear a smacking sound, it is a poor latch and the baby should be removed from the nipple to relatch. Show and encourage the mom to place a washed finger in the corner of the infant's mouth to break the suck seal; otherwise, significant damage can be done to the nipple. An immediate benefit is it reduces the risk of postpartum hemorrhage (PPH) because it aids in UCX.

Colostrum is present in the first few days after birth. It contains proteins, vitamins, minerals, potassium, sodium, IgA, IgG, and IgM from the mom. It also works as a laxative to help the infant pass all the meconium and protects against viruses and bacteria. There is no substitute for the colostrum, which gives the infant its mother's immunities.

Benefits of Breastfeeding—This list is not all inclusive.

- Decreases both the mother's and the infant's risk for certain cancers later in life
- Decreases the infant's risk for childhood and adult obesity
- More quickly returns mother to prepregnancy weight
- Builds up infant's defense against bacteria and viruses
- Decreases mother's risk for postpartum depression
- Decreases the risk of necrotizing enterocolitis, or NEC, and asthma in the infant
- Decreases infant risk of cavities and ear infections

Positions

- Cradle hold: Across the mother's abdomen, easiest for first-time mothers
- Football hold: Infant lies by the mother's side supported in her arm
- Side lying: Mother is on her side and infant is supported by the bed. More difficult position for new mothers

Latch

- The infant's mouth should be wide open.
- The lower lip should make first contact with breast.
- The infant should grasp both the areola and the entire nipple (never just the nipple).
- Smacking sounds are indicative of a poor latch.

Contraindications to Breastfeeding

- Mothers who are HIV positive or who have TB
- Mothers taking certain prescribed drugs

Lactation Drug Categories

A	Safe	Studied on humans
B	Presumed safe	Studied on animals
C		No studies available
D	Unsafe	Studies have shown adverse effects on infant
X	Contraindicated	Should not be used

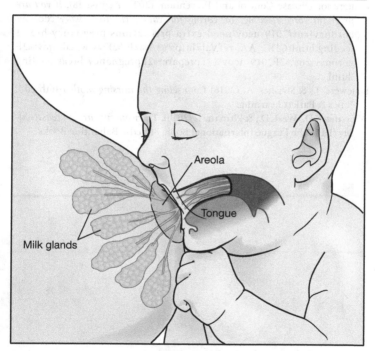

Proper Latch

Fast Fact

At the time of this printing, the Centers for Disease Control and Prevention (CDC) recommends that COVID-19–positive mothers who choose to breastfeed should frequently wash their hands and wear a mask when around the newborn. Mothers may also choose to express or pump breast milk for their babies. COVID-19 is not a contraindication for breastfeeding.

Sources

Centers for Disease Control and Prevention. (2021, August 18). *If you are pregnant, breastfeeding, or caring for young children.* www.cdc.gov/ coronavirus/2019-ncov/need-extra-precautions/pregnancy-breast feeding.html?CDC_AA_refVal=https%3A%2F%2Fwww. cdc.gov%2F coronavirus%2F2019-ncov%2Fprepare%2Fpregnancy-breastfeeding .html

Lauewers, J., & Swisher, A. (2016) *Counseling the nursing mother* (6th ed.). Jones & Barlett Learning.

Wiessinger, D., West, D., & Pitman, T. (2010). *The womanly art of breastfeeding* (La Leche League International Book; 8th ed.). Ballantine Books.

CERVIX IN LABOR

Dilatation

0 to 10 cm

- First stage of labor
    - 0- to 3-cm latent phase of labor
        - Primip average length — 6.5 hr
        - Multip average length — 5 hr
    - 4- to 7-cm active phase of labor
        - Primip average length — 4.5 hr
        - Multip average length — 2.5 hr
    - 8- to 10-cm transition phase of labor
        - Primip average length — 3.5 hr
        - Multip average length — Varies
- Second stage of labor—10 cm to delivery
    - Primip average length — 3 hr
    - Multip average length — 0 to 30 min
- Third stage of labor—birth to delivery of placenta
    - 0 to 30 min

Effacement

- Refers to the length of cervix between 0% and 100%

There is research that suggests labor progression based on Friedman's curve is not accurate. In fact, the active phase of labor may not begin until 5 cm or greater depending on the individual woman. Some factors that can influence when active labor begins are body mass index, ethnicity, and parity. Remember the definition of *labor*: regular uterine contractions that cause cervical dilatation.

Cervical Ripening
Bishop score can predict success of the induction.

Adverse Effects
- Hyperstimulation
- Nonreassuring fetal heart rate (FHR)
- Failed induction

Contraindications
- Prior uterine surgery

- Preterm
- Malposition of fetus, for example, breech or transverse
- Unexplained vaginal bleeding
- Maternal infection or fever of unknown origin

Medications for Cervical Ripening

- Dinoprostone (Cervidil) 10 mg PV q 12 hr. Patient must stay in bed for 2 hr after insertion
- Dinoprostone (Prepidil) .5 mg PV q 6 hr max 3 doses
- Misoprostol (Cytotec) 25 to 50 mcg PV q 3 to 4 hr

Nonpharmacological Cervical Ripening

- Stripping membranes
- Transcervical Foley balloon (Cook's balloon): inflating a Foley balloon in cervix to dilate

What You Need for Foley Balloon Insertion

- 24 French Foley catheter
- Syringe
- 30 mL of sterile water
- Sterile gloves
- Speculum
- Tenaculum
- Ring forceps
- Pack of 2 x 2 s
- Betadine
- Sterile field

Sources

American College of Obstetricians and Gynecologists. (2009). ACOG Practice Bulletin No. 107: Induction of labor. *Obstetrics & Gynecology, 114* (Issue 2, Pt. 1), 386–397. https://doi.org/10.1097/AOG.0b013e3181b48ef5

Chou, B., Bienstock, J. L., & Satin, A. J. (2021). *The Johns Hopkins manual of gynecology and obstetrics* (6th ed.). Wolters Kluwer Health.

Epocrates. (2020). www.epocrates.com

CESAREAN SECTION (C/S)

Circulating RN's Responsibility

Preparation for C/S

- Admission of patient to L&D
- IV 18G (if patient has 20G IV placed, you have to change to 18G before going to the OR)
- Obtaining laboratory reports (type and screen should be drawn within 72 hours of C/S)
- Citric acid/sodium citrate (Bicitra) administration if ordered
- Blood bank type and crossmatch 2 units on standby
- Documenting fetal heart rate (FHR)

In OR

- Verify patient ID, surgery, and physician doing surgery
- Check all equipment (infant warmer, O2, suction)
- Position for anesthesia
- Apply compression boots
- Insert Foley catheter
- Place electrode pad on thigh
- *First count with scrub tech*
- Drape patient
- Suction hookup
- Electrosurgery hookup
- Notify pediatrician for C/S delivery
- Count after
  - Uterus is closed
  - Fascia closed
  - Skin is closed
- Verify estimated blood loss
- Verify Apgar
- Assist moving patient from the OR table to recovery room

General Instruments

Ring forceps	4
T-clamps	8
Allis clamps	4
Kochers	4
Curved Kellys	6
Straight Halsteds	6

Tube occluding forceps	5
Lap sponges	20
Bovie tip	1
Blades	2
Needles	Depends on surgeon
Needle holders	4
Towel clips	4
Scissors	4
Forceps	4
Scalpels	2
Self-retaining retractors	6
Suction tips	2

Note: Numbers may vary by institution.

Sources

Maternity Center. (2007, April 11). *Maternity center circulating for cesarean delivery* [Unpublished procedure manual]. Overlook Hospital Department of OB/GYN.

Schaarschmidt, D. (2009, March 9). Charge nurse St. Barnabas Medical Center. Personal Interview.

DATING A PREGNANCY (ASSESSMENT FOR GESTATIONAL AGE)

You may see estimated due date (EDD) or estimated date of confinement (EDC); both are acceptable abbreviations.

Naegele's Rule
If patient is sure of LMP,
    LMP – 3 Months + 7 Days + 1 Year = EDC

Ultrasound
- What is measured:
  - Biparietal diameter
  - Head circumference
  - Femoral diaphysis length
  - Abdominal circumference
  - Estimated fetal weight
- Most accurate in first trimester
- Second trimester can be inaccurate by 1 to 2 weeks
- Third trimester can be inaccurate by 2 to 3 weeks

  If there is a discrepancy between U/S and LMP:

- First trimester: Use the U/S EDC if the discrepancy is greater than 7 days.
- Second trimester: Use the U/S EDC if the discrepancy is greater than 10 days.

Blood work	Beta-hCG (human chorionic gonadotropin) levels
3–4 wk	150–1,000 mLU/mL
4–5 wk	greater than 1,000–2,000 mLU/mL
5–6 wk	1,000–7,200 mLU/mL
6–7 wk	greater than 10,800 mLU/mL

Less Accurate Ways to Measure (No Clinical Diagnosis Should Be Made Based on Findings)
If the patient does not know her LMP and no U/S is available, you can measure with tape measure or index finger.

Tape Measure
Using centimeter side of tape, measure from pubic symphysis to fundus.

No Tape Measure
Start at umbilicus and measure to top of fundus using the width of your index finger. Start at number 20 and count every finger width as 1 cm. Each finger width or centimeter is equal to 1 gestational week.

Rule of Thumb

- 16 weeks + halfway between umbilicus and pubic symphysis
- 20 weeks = at umbilicus

Factors That Influence Uterine Size in Pregnancy

- Full bladder
- Amniotic fluid index
- Fibroids
- Multiple gestations
- Fetal position
- Large-for-gestational age/small-for-gestational age
- Maternal weight
- Fetal anomalies

Sources

Committee on Practice Bulletins—Obstetrics and the American Institute of Ultrasound in Medicine. (2016). Practice Bulletin No. 175: Ultrasound in pregnancy. *Obstetrics & Gynecology, 128*(6), e241–e256. https://doi.org/10.10197/AOG.0000000000001815

King, T., Brucker, M., Osborne, K., & Jevitt, C.M. (2018). *Varney's midwifery* (6th ed.). Sudbury, MA: Jones & Bartlett Learning.

DRUG CLASSIFICATIONS

In Pregnancy

A	Controlled studies of pregnant women do not show any adverse effects on fetus.
B	Animal studies have shown no adverse effects on fetus, but no controlled study has been performed on pregnant women.
C	There are no studies either on animals or pregnant women showing adverse effect on fetus.
D	Studies on pregnant women did exhibit an adverse effect on fetus. In certain diagnoses, benefits of medication use may outweigh the risks.
X	This is contraindicated for women who may attempt or are attempting to become pregnant.

In Lactation

L_1	Safest	There is no evidence of adverse effects to infant and does not affect the mother's milk supply in large studies.
L_2	Safer	There is no evidence of adverse effects to infant and does not affect the mother's milk supply in limited studies.
L_3	Moderately safe	Either no study or effects were minimal with no risk to infant
L_4	Possibly hazardous	There is a risk to nursing infant or to the production of milk supply.
L_5	Contraindicated	There is a significant risk to infant or to milk production and use should be avoided.

Sources

Briggs, G. G., & Freedman, R. K. (2014). *Drugs in pregnancy and lactation* (10th ed.). Lippincott Williams & Wilkins.
Epocrates. (2020). www.epocrates.com
Hale, T. W. (2018). *Hale's medications & mothers' milk* (18th ed.). Springer.
Perinatology.com. (2020). *FDA use-in-pregnancy ratings.* www.perinatology .com/exposures/Drugs/FDACategories.htm

ELECTRONIC FETAL MONITORING (EFM)

Three categories for defining and interpreting FHR are as follows:

Category I

- Normal tracing
  - FHR between 110 and 160
- Moderate variability (beat-to-beat variability is between 6 and 25 bpm)
- Accelerations and early decelerations may or may not be present
- No late or variable decelerations

Category II

> **Fast Fact**
>
> Continuous EFM—notify physician or midwife.

- Uncertain tracing
  - Marked variability
- Absent variability without recurrent late or variable decelerations
- Tachycardia
- Bradycardia without variability or with minimal variability
- Periodic decelerations
- Recurrent variables without variability or with minimal variability
- Deceleration greater than 2 minutes but less than 10 minutes
- No acceleration after fetal scalp stimulation

Category III

> **Fast Fact**
>
> Abnormal tracing—contact physician or midwife immediately and notify senior nurses.

- Recurrent late or variable decelerations
- Bradycardia
- Sinusoidal pattern

Definitions

Baseline	FHR between 110 and 160	
Tachycardia	FHR more than 160	mostly seen with maternal fever
Bradycardia	FHR less than 110	mostly seen in compromised fetus

Variability

Minimal	0–5 bpm	may be fetus sleep cycle; continue to monitor
Moderate	6–25 bpm	reassuring
Marked	greater than 25 bpm	may be a sign of fetal hypoxia

Acceleration—FHR 15 bpm above baseline for 15 seconds or greater (longer than 10 minutes is change in baseline)
   Deceleration—FHR below the baseline

- Early—nadir of deceleration with peak of contraction (present with pushing or head compression)
- Late—deceleration begins immediately after peak of contraction (recurrent is ominous sign)
- Variable—usually V-shaped and may occur at any time. May correlate with cord compression

Reactive FHR is when two accelerations are noted within a 10-minute period.

Sinusoidal—undulating pattern with no baseline or variability able to be appreciated. Usually 3 to 5 cycles/min. Notify the physician or midwife immediately. Seen mostly when a fetus is severely compromised.

Contractions

- Tectonic: resting tone greater than 30 mmHg or firm uterus by palpation
- Tachysystole: more than five contractions in a 10-minute period or contraction lasting greater than 90 seconds
- Intensity can only be measured with IUPC

Internal Fetal Monitoring (IFM)

ISE—electrode that is attached to fetal scalp. Most accurate way to assess FHR. Membranes must be ruptured and the patient must be 2 to 3 cm dilated.

What You Need

- Sterile gloves
- ISE lead and connecting wire

- Tape (to tape lead to patient's leg)
- Amnihook if needed for AROM
- FHR will sound like a "ping" when working appropriately

IUPC—catheter is inserted and lies next to fetus to measure pressure of contractions within the uterus. This is the only way to document accurate uterine resting tone and intensity. Membranes must be ruptured and patient must be 2 to 3 cm dilated.

What You Need
- Sterile gloves
- IUPC lead and connecting wire
- Tape (to tape lead to patient's leg)
- After first contraction, zero out the IUPC to assess accurate resting tone
- Amnihook if needed for AROM

Documentation
- Baseline EHR
- Variability
- Accelerations and decelerations present
- Contractions
- EFM versus ISE
- Toco versus IUPC
- Notification of physician or midwife
- Intervention and outcome

Intrauterine Resuscitation

Nonreassuring Tracing
- Stop induction agent, for example, oxytocin (Pitocin) or remove dinoprostone (Cervidil).
- Give 10 L/min of O2 through facemask.
- Increase IV fluids.
- Change maternal position.
- Anticipate possible amnioinfusion.
- Be sure to alert other nurses that you may need help and always use closed-loop communication.
- Notify physician or midwife.

Tachysystole
- Stop induction agent, for example, oxytocin (Pitocin), or remove dinoprostone (Cervidil).
- Increase IV fluids.
- Anticipate tocolytics to be given (e.g., Terbutaline .25 mg SQ).
- Notify physician or midwife.

Hypotension (Maternal)

- Lay patient flat.
- Increase IV fluids.
- Anticipate ephedrine 5- to 10-mg IV push (not for RN administration).
- Notify anesthetist and physician or midwife.

Sources

American College of Obstetricians and Gynecologists. (2009). Intrapartum fetal heart rate monitoring: Nomenclature, interpretation, and general management principles (Practice Bulletin No. 106). In *2009 compendium of selected publications* (pp. 192–202).

Chou, B., Bienstock, J. L., & Satin, A. J. (2021). *The Johns Hopkins manual of gynecology and obstetrics* (6th ed.). Wolters Kluwer Health.

Simpson, K. R., & Creehan, P. A. (2021). *AWHONN perinatal nursing* (5th ed.). Wolters Kluwer Health.

EMERGENCY DRUGS

Indication	Drug name–generic (trade)	Dosage, route, and frequency	Comments/cautions
Preterm labor			
Corticosteroids (for fetal lung maturity)			
	Betamethasone (Celestone)	12 mg IM q 12 hr × 2 doses	
	Dexamethasone	6 mg IM q 12 hr × 4 doses	
Tocolytics (to try to stop labor)			
	Indomethacin (Indocin)	50–100 mg PO at first dose, then 25–50 mg PO q 4–6 hr	Do not give if oligohydramnios
	Nifedipine (Procardia)	10–20 mg PO q 6 hr	
	Terbutaline	.25 mg SQ q 20–30 min PRN	May cause maternal tachycardia
	Magnesium sulfate (MgSO4)	Loading dose: 4–6 g IV, then 2–4 g IV/hr	Serum magnesium (Mg) level should be drawn q 6 hr
			Levels should be between 6 and 8 mg/dL
			Levels 8–10 mg/dL + decrease deep tendon reflexes
			Levels 13–15 mg/dL + respiratory distress
			Levels >15 mg/dL + cardiac arrest
			Monitor I&O
			Manage IV drip so no more than 125 mL/hr infuses
			Antidote: calcium gluconate 1 g IV over 3 min
Postpartum hemorrhage			
	Oxytocin (Pitocin)	10 IU/mL IM or 40 U IV	Should have drug in room at every delivery
	Methylergonovine (Methergine)	.2 mg IM q 2–4 hr	Do not give hypertension (HTN)/preeclamptic patients
			Keep in refrigerator

Indication	Drug name–generic (trade)	Dosage, route, and frequency	Comments/cautions
	Carboprost (Hemabate)	250 mcg IM q 15–90 min; maximum 8 doses	Do not give with history of asthma
Preeclampsia			
	Magnesium sulfate	Loading dose: 4–6 g IV, then 2–4 g IV/hr	Serum magnesium (Mg) level should be drawn q 6 hr
			Levels should be between 6 and 8 mg/dL
			Levels 8–10 mg/dL + decrease deep tendon reflexes
			Levels 13–15 mg/dL + respiratory distress
			Levels >15 mg/dL + cardiac arrest
			Monitor I&O
			Manage IV drip so no more than 125 mL/hr infuses
			Antidote: calcium gluconate 1 g IV over 3 min
	Labetalol (Trandate)	20 mg IV push then increase dose at 10 min intervals to 20, 40, 80 mg, for max 300 mg/24 hr	NOT FOR RN ADMINISTRATION
	Hydralazine	5 mg IV bolus q 20 min until 20 mg PRN	
Opioid-addicted mother (for nonresponsive or low-Apgar neonate)			
	Nalozone	.1 mg/kg IV, IM, or SQ, q 2–3 min PRN	Pediatrician should be at delivery

Fast Fact

Antidote for hypermagnesemia: calcium gluconate 1 g IV over 3 minutes; should be in room if MgSO4 is infusing.

Sources

Cunningham, G., & Leveno, K. J. (2018). *Williams obstetrics* (25th ed.). McGraw-Hill.

Epocrates. (2020). www.epocrates.com

American College of Obstetricians and Gynecologists' Committee on Practice Bulletins—Obstetrics. (2016). ACOG Practice Bulletin No. 171: Management of preterm labor. *Obstetrics and Gynecology, 128*, e155–e164. https://doi.org/10.1097/AOG.0000000000001711

Simpson, K. R., & Creehan, P. A. (2021). *AWHONN perinatal nursing* (5th ed.). Wolters Kluwer Health.

FETAL DEMISE (INTRAUTERINE FETAL DEATH [IUFD])

Cardiac activity is not noted by real-time U/S after 20 weeks, often referred to as stillborn.

If possible, take infant warmer out of room before patient is admitted to room. Place a sign (often a picture) indicating that there is a fetal demise so that other personnel on the unit are aware.

What to Do

- Proceed as with induction
- Admit to L&D
- IV access
- Admission labs
- Toco (ONLY)
- Vital signs (VS)
- Patient history

Depending on Bishop score and gestational age, the determination of appropriate medication should be ordered by the physician or midwife.

Most Often Ordered Induction Agents

- Misoprostol (Cytotec)
- Oxytocin (Pitocin)

What to Expect

- Delivery is often quick once patient has dilated.
- Placenta delivery may take longer than 30 minutes.
- Be prepared, be sensitive, and be professional.

What to Do

- Wrap the baby and offer to mother.
- Save the baby hat, take photos and footprints, and put all in memory box.
- Give supportive care as needed.
- Contact a social worker and/or pastoral care (as appropriate).

Fast Fact

The organization Now I Lay Me Down to Sleep provides families with free professional photography sessions. If a photographer is available in your area, the family should be informed and given the option.

I was told many times in my training to never cry in front of a patient, that it is unprofessional. I have never found a more appropriate time to cry than witnessing the death of someone's child. It has never impeded my ability to do my job, and a family member has never called me unprofessional for genuinely grieving with them. You entered this profession because you are compassionate; sometimes you will find it will be all you have left to offer and that may be all the patient and their family need.

Sources

Maternity Center. (2010, March 10). *Maternity center induction of labor for fetal demise/nonviable fetus* [Unpublished procedure manual]. Overlook Hospital Department of OB/GYN.

Now I Lay Me Down to Sleep. (2011). www.nowilaymedowntosleep.org

FETAL KICK COUNTS

Used to assess the well-being of the fetus. The test is subjective and performed by the mother.

Process for Conducting the Test
- Done after 28 weeks gestation.
- Have the mother lie on her left side.
- Instruct her to count the number of kicks or movements she feels within 2 hours.

Interpretation of the Test
- Reassuring if more than 10 movements are counted.
- The patient should call her provider immediately or come to L&D for assessment if fewer than 10 are counted or if no movements are felt.
- If the patient states she has felt no fetal movement for 24 hours, she should be seen immediately.

Sources
Cunningham, G., & Leveno, K. J. (2018). *Williams obstetrics* (25th ed.). McGraw-Hill.

King, T., Brucker, M., Osborne, K., & Jevitt, C. M. (2018). *Varney's midwifery* (6th ed.). Jones & Bartlett Learning.

GESTATIONAL DIABETES MELLITUS (GDM)

Usually diagnosed between 16 and 28 weeks of pregnancy, depending on maternal risk factor.

Maternal Complications

- DKA
- Preeclampsia
- Preterm labor and delivery

Fetal Complications

- Congenital malformation
- Polyhydramnios
- Macrosomia
- Intrauterine growth restriction (IUGR)
- Fetal demise
- Shoulder dystocia
- Neonatal hypoglycemia

Management

- Patients may be induced between 39 and 40 weeks.
- For patients with EFW greater than 4,500 g, C/S delivery is indicated and should be offered to the patient.
- Prepare room for shoulder dystocia for anticipated NSVD (extra staff members, foot stool medications for postpartum hemorrhage).

Management on L&D

- Normal saline IV
- Finger stick: q hour until stable (between 70 and 110 mg/dL)
    - q 2 hr until delivery
- Notify MD if glucose is less than 60 or greater than 150 mg/dL
- Monitor hourly I&Os
- Continuous fetal monitoring

What You Need for an Insulin Drip

(*USUALLY NOT FOR PATIENTS WHO HAVE TYPE 2 OR GDM*)

- Infusion pump
- Insulin is ALWAYS intravenous piggy-back (IVPB) to primary IV of normal saline
- Prime IV tubing with at least 50 mL of insulin solution before starting infusion
- Insulin drip is 100 units of regular insulin in 100 mL of normal saline
- Follow orders and institutional protocol for rate
- Discontinue drip at time of delivery

Hypoglycemia Clinical Presentation

- Blood sugar less than 60 mg/dL
- Nausea
- Headache
- Diaphoresis
- Visual changes
- Weakness
- Confusion

What to Do for Hypoglycemia

- Notify the MD immediately
- If no IV, give 4 ounces of juice
- If you have an IV, start D5NS at 12 mL/hr
- Repeat finger stick q 15 min until BS above 70 mg/dL

Diabetic Ketoacidosis (DKA)

Not enough circulating insulin in the body to metabolize glucose.

Clinical Presentation

- Abdominal pain
- Nausea
- Vomiting
- Hypotension
- Tachypnea
- Confusion
- Lethargy
- Sweet-smelling breath

What to Do

- Call the physician STAT
- Call the anesthetist STAT
- EKG STAT
- Blood gases STAT (may need to call respiratory to obtain)
- Labs: CMP, acetone, and ketone bodies STAT and then q 1 to 2 hr
- 18G IV started with normal saline bolus 1 L over 30 min
- Give O2 8 to 10 L/min through face mask
- EFM continuous
- Pulse oximetry continuous
- Anticipate: Intubation
  - Insulin infusion as per physician orders
  - Sodium bicarbonate as ordered if pH is <7.1
- Monitor for signs of pulmonary edema
  - Hypovolemia
  - Cerebral edema

Fast Fact

Antenatal steroids and tocolytics can cause or worsen DKA.

Sources

American College of Obstetricians and Gynecologists' Committee on Practice Bulletins—Obstetrics. (2018). ACOG Practice Bulletin No. 190: Gestational diabetes mellitus. *Obstetrics & Gynecology, 131,* e49–e64. https://doi.org/10.1097/AOG.0000000000002501

American College of Obstetricians and Gynecologists' Committee on Practice Bulletins—Obstetrics. (2018). ACOG Practice Bulletin No. 201: Pregestational diabetes mellitus. *Obstetrics & Gynecology, 132,* e228–e248. https://doi.org/10.1097/AOG.0000000000002960

Chou, B., Bienstock, J. L., & Satin, A. J. (2021). *The Johns Hopkins manual of gynecology and obstetrics* (6th ed.). Wolters Kluwer Health.

Cunningham, G., & Leveno, K. J. (2018). *Williams obstetrics* (25th ed.). McGraw-Hill.

GROUP B *STREPTOCOCCUS* (GBS)

A gram-positive bacterium that colonizes in the vagina, urethra, and/or rectum and can cause premature birth/premature rupture of membranes (PROM), sepsis, pneumonia, and meningitis. A swab should be obtained at 35 to 37 weeks. If results were negative and patient delivers 5 weeks after initial GBS screening, consider obtaining another swab.

2020 Guidelines

Intrapartum (IP) GBS prophylaxis indicated	IP GBS prophylaxis not indicated
Previous infant with invasive GBS disease	Colonization with GBS during a previous pregnancy (unless an indication for GBS prophylaxis is present for current pregnancy)
GBS bacteriuria during any trimester of the current pregnancy	GBS bacteriuria during previous pregnancy (unless an indication for GBS prophylaxis is present for current pregnancy)
Positive GBS vaginal–rectal screening culture in late gestation during current pregnancy	Negative vaginal and rectal GBS screening culture in late gestation during the current pregnancy, regardless of IP risk factors
Unknown GBS status at the onset of labor (culture not done, incomplete, or results unknown) and any of the following: Delivery at <37 wk gestation • Amniotic membrane rupture +18 hr • IP temperature +38 °C • IP NAAT positive for GBS	Cesarean delivery performed before onset of labor on a woman with intact amniotic membranes, regardless of GBS colonization status or gestational age

GBS, Group B Streptococcus; NAAT, nucleic acid amplification tests.
Source: Centers for Disease Control and Prevention (2010).
Prevention of group B streptococcal early-onset disease in newborns. ACOG Committee Opinion No. 797. American College of Obstetricians and Gynecologists. Obstet Gynecol 2020;135:e51–72.

Treatment in Preterm Labor

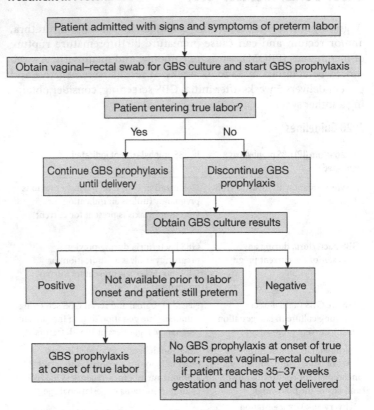

Source: Centers for Disease Control and Prevention (2010).

If patient has PPROM, swab and treat for 48 hours.

Treatment in Labor

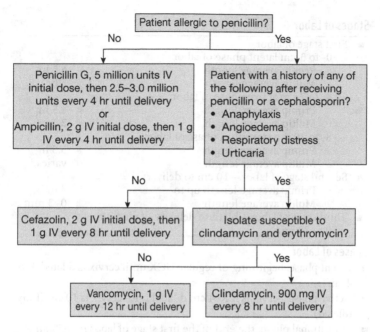

Source: Centers for Disease Control and Prevention (2010).

Source

Prevention of group B streptoccical early-onset disease in newborns. (2020). ACOG Committee Opinion No. 797. *Obstetricians and Gynecologists, 135,* e51–e72.

LABOR PROGRESSION

Stages of Labor

- First stage of labor
  - 0- to 3-cm latent phase of labor
    - Primip average length
    - Multip average length
  - 4- to 7-cm active phase of labor
    - Primip average length
    - Multip average length
  - 8- to 10-cm transition phase of labor
    - Primip average length
    - Multip average length
- Second stage of labor—10 cm to delivery
    - Primip average length up to
    - Multip average length
- Third stage of labor—birth to delivery of placenta
  - 0 to 30 min

Primip average length	6.5 hr
Multip average length	5 hr
Primip average length	4.5 hr
Multip average length	2.5 hr
Primip average length	3.5 hr
Multip average length	varies
Primip average length up to	3 hr
Multip average length	0–3 min

Phases of Labor

- Latent phase: beginning of regular UCX until cervix is dilated 3 to 4 cm
- Active phase: cervix is 3 to 4 cm dilated until cervix is 10 cm (fully dilated)
- Transitional phase: the end of the first stage of labor *transitioning* into the second stage of labor

As stated earlier, there is research regarding exactly when the active phase of labor begins. Studies are showing that active labor often begins later than 4 cm and every patient should be evaluated on an individual basis. The definitions of the phases, as of now, have not changed.

Dystocia of Labor

- Premature rupture of membranes: ROM prior to the onset of labor
- Arrest of labor (failure of descent or failure to progress): at least 4 cm, adequate UCX (200–225 MVU), and no cervical dilatation in 4 hr

Sources

American College of Obstetricians and Gynecologists' Committee on Obstetric Practice. (2017). ACOG Committee Opinion No. 766: Approaches to limited intervention during labor and birth. *Obstetrics & Gynecology, 133*, e164–e173. https://doi.org/10.1097/AOG.0000000000003074

American College of Obstetricians and Gynecologists. (2020). ACOG Committee Opinion No. 797: Prevention of group B streptococcal early onset disease in newborns. *Obstetrics & Gynecology, 135*, e51–e72. https://doi.org/10.1097/AOG.0000000000003668

King, T., Brucker, M., Osborne, K., & Jevitt, C. M. (2018). *Varney's midwifery* (6th ed.). Jones & Bartlett Learning.

Simpson, K. R., & Creehan, P. A. (2021). *AWHONN perinatal nursing* (5th ed.). Wolters Kluwer Health.

LABS

Skeletons/Fishbones

The correct format to represent your laboratory values in a paper chart.

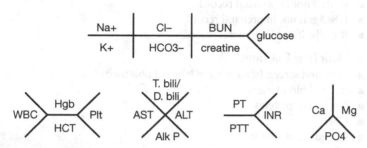

Fast Fact

If at any time a patient may need to have a C/S, the blood bank should be called and 2 units should be crossmatched and readily available. The refrigerator in unit should also have O-negative (emergency release) blood and should be checked to ensure it is not expired at the beginning of every shift.

Abdominal Trauma
- Type and screen
- Antibody screen
- Crossmatch (if patient may need C/S)
- CBC
- KB
- Coagulation profile
- Toxicology

Abruptio Placentae
- CBC
- Type and screen
- PT/PTT
- Fibrinogen
- Fibrin split products
- Toxicology

Admission Labs to L&D

- CBC
- Urine dipstick
- Blood type and Rh
- Antibody screen
- RPR: if not in prenatal record
- HBsAg: if not in prenatal record
- Rubella: if not in prenatal record

Amniotic Fluid Embolism

- Type and screen (if admission labs not obtained)
- Arterial blood gases
- Serum electrolytes
- CMP
- Coagulation profile
- CBC

Preeclampsia

- CBC
- Liver function panel
- Kidney function panel
- PT/PTT
- Fibrinogen
- Urine dipstick/urinalysis
- 24-hour urine collection

Sources

Chou, B., Bienstock, J. L., & Satin, A. J. (2021). *The Johns Hopkins manual of gynecology and obstetrics* (6th ed.). Wolters Kluwer Health.

Cunningham, G., & Leveno, K. J. (2018). *Williams obstetrics* (25th ed.). McGraw-Hill.

American College of Obstetricians and Gynecologists. (2020). ACOG Practice Bulletin No. 222: Gestational hypertension and preeclampsia. *Obstetrics & Gynecology, 135*, e237–e260. https://doi.org/10.1097/AOG.0000000000003891

MAGNESIUM SULFATE (MgSO4)

Used for preeclampsia/eclampsia and preterm labor (PTL). The drug affects the central nervous system (CNS) and functions as a smooth muscle relaxer and anticonvulsant.

In the use of magnesium sulfate for preeclampsia/eclampsia, the drug is given as an anticonvulsant, not for hypertension. A side effect is a decrease in blood pressure (BP), but this may be temporary and have a rebound effect. Continue monitoring BP and notify the practitioner if it exceeds parameters.

Magnesium sulfate will not work for PTL if the patient is in active labor.

Side Effects
- Flushing
- Muscle weakness
- Blurred vision
- Headache
- Lethargy
- Nausea/vomiting
- Bradycardia
- Respiratory depression

Contraindications
- Respiratory depression
- Systolic BP less than 110
- Heart block
- Myasthenia gravis

Administration
- Magnesium sulfate
  - Loading dose 4 to 6 g IV
  - Maintenance 2 to 4 g IV/hr
  - Serum Mg level should be drawn q 6 hr
  - Levels should be between 6 and 8 mg/dL
- Serum Mg levels
  - 5 to 9 mg/dL therapeutic
  - Greater than 9 mg/dL decrease deep tendon reflexes
  - Greater than 12 mg/dL respiratory paralysis
  - Greater than 30 mg/dL cardiac arrest

Monitor I&Os; IV fluid needs to be managed so no more than 125 mL/hr of total IV fluid is infusing.

Fast Fact

Antidote to hypermagnesemia: calcium gluconate 1 g IV over 3 minutes; should be in room if MgSO4 is infusing.

Sources

Chou, B., Bienstock, J. L., & Satin, A. J. (2021). *The Johns Hopkins manual of gynecology and obstetrics* (6th ed.). Wolters Kluwer Health.

Epocrates. (2020). www.epocrates.com

American College of Obstetricians and Gynecologists. (2020). ACOG Practice Bulletin No. 222: Gestational hypertension and preeclampsia. *Obstetrics & Gynecology, 135,* e237–260. https://doi.org/10.1097/AOG .0000000000003891

MONTEVIDEO UNITS (MVU)

Measures the intensity of UCX and diagnoses their adequacy for labor. Can be done only when an IUPC is in place.

What You Need for IUPC Placement
- Amnihook if needed for AROM
- Sterile gloves
- IUPC lead and connecting wire
- Tape (to tape lead to patient's leg)
- After first contraction, zero out the IUPC to assess accurate resting tone

To Calculate MVU
Take the contraction strength of each contraction occurring within a 10-minute period and add the intensity together.

To Calculate Intensity of UCX
Take the baseline uterine pressure and subtract it from the peak height of the contraction.

Example intensity calculation: Uterine resting tone is at 20 mmHg; the peak of that UCX is 100 mmHg.

100 mmHg	UCX intensity = 80 mmHg
−20 mmHg	
80 mmHg	

Example MVU calculation: Patient has 3 UCX in 10 minutes each with the following intensity.

80 mmHg	MVU = 225
75 mmHg	
+70 mmHg	
225 mmHg	

Sources
Cunningham, G., & Leveno, K. J. (2018). *Williams obstetrics* (25th ed.). McGraw-Hill.

Maternity Center. (2010, June 9). *Maternity center: Intrauterine pressure catheter* [Unpublished procedure manual]. Overlook Hospital Department of OB/GYN.

MULTIPLE GESTATIONS

A pregnancy in which more than one fetus is conceived at the same time. Can be spontaneous or because of infertility treatment. Most facilities allow cephalic/cephalic to try NSVD; however, if cephalic/breech a C/S is usually performed. Most vaginal twins are delivered in the OR.

Risks/Complications

- PTL/delivery
- IUGR
- Preeclampsia
- Postpartum hemorrhage
- Gestational diabetes
- Twin-to-twin transfusion
- Cord accident (monochromic/monoamniotic)
- Increased occurrence of C/S
- Placental abnormalities

Types of Multiple Gestations

	Approximate occurrence (%)	Placenta	Amniotic sac
Dizygotic/ Dichorionic/ diamnionic (fraternal)	75	2	2
Monozygotic (identical)	25	Varies depending on time of cleavage	Varies depending on time of cleavage
Dichorionic/diamnionic Monozygotic	8	2	2
Monochorionic/ diamnionic	17	1 fused	2
Monochorionic/ monoamnionic	<1	1	1

Always make sure you have two different heartbeats when monitoring twins. Sometimes they can be very similar and frustrating. Placing a pulse Ox on the mother may help rule out that you are not recording her heart rate instead of one of the twins.

Sources

Chou, B., Bienstock, J. L., Satin, A. J. (2021). *The Johns Hopkins manual of gynecology and obstetrics* (6th ed.). Wolters Kluwer Health.

King, T., Brucker, M., Osborne, K., & Jevitt, C. M. (2018). *Varney's midwifery* (6th ed.). Jones & Bartlett Learning.

NEWBORN

If possible, always place the baby on the mother immediately after delivery. The infant can be cleaned, wrapped in a blanket or skin-to-skin, VS taken, and ID bands placed all while on the mother's chest.

Room Setup
- Ensure access to all the mother's antenatal blood work
- Warmer
- Blankets
- Oxygen
- Suction
- Diaper
- Infant hat
- Laryngoscope
- Umbilical cord clamp
- Scissors
- Thermometer
- Infant pulsometer
- Erythromycin ophthalmic ointment .5% *(administered in newborn's eyes for prophylaxis against GC/CT)*
- Vitamin K (phytonadione) 1 mg IM × 1 dose *(administered in newborns for prophylaxis of classic hemorrhagic disease)*

What to Do
- Assess the newborn (if at any point the Apgars are less than 7, notify pediatrician STAT)
- Place ID bands on mother and infant
- Document time of birth and placenta delivery
- Obtain cord blood
- Assist the mother in breastfeeding

Sources

King, T., Brucker, M., Osborne, K., & Jevitt, C. M. (2018). *Varney's midwifery* (6th ed.). Jones & Bartlett Learning.

Simpson, K. R., & Creehan, P. A. (2021). *AWHONN perinatal nursing* (5th ed.). Wolters Kluwer Health.

PAIN MANAGEMENT

Distraction Methods
- Guided imagery
- Music
- Focal points
- Relaxation techniques
- Breathing techniques

Positions That Most Commonly Relieve Pressure and Discomfort
- Walking
- Swaying
- Sitting on toilet
- Leaning over back of bed (raise the back of the hospital bed to upright position; the mother kneels on bed)
- Squatting
- Lying on her side
- Sitting on a birthing ball

Interventions to Relieve Back Pain
- Ice packs to lower back
- Getting into shower with water directed to lower back
- Getting into bathtub
- Counterpressure (someone places their fists on the mother's lower back and presses hard during contraction)

Most Common IV Medication

Phenergan is often given to potentiate the effects of pain medication; however, it is extremely caustic and should be used with caution and be administered only in a diluted solution to prevent phlebitis or other vascular injury.

Use caution when administering IV pain medication. IV pain medication should be administered only if the delivery time is anticipated to be more than 4 hours from the time of administration to avoid possible respiratory depression in the neonate.

Fast Fact

The patient should not be ambulatory after medication is administered.

Pain Medication

Nalbuphine (Nubain)	5–10 mg	q 4 hr PRN
Morphine	1–2 mg	q 4 hr PRN
Butorphanol (Stadol)	1–2 mg	q 4 hr PRN
Meperidine (Demerol)	25–50 mg	q 4 hr PRN
Promethazine (Phenergan) (also used for nausea in labor)	12.5–25 mg	q 4 hr PRN

Side Effects
- Lethargy
- Respiratory depression for the mother and neonate
- Disorientation
- Pruritus
- Hypotension

Local Anesthesia

Lidocaine injection lasts approximately 20 to 40 minutes and gives relief for the cutting episiotomies and repairing vaginal laceration. Pudendal block allows for pain relief during a vaginal delivery due to numbing effects of lidocaine being injected into the pudendal nerve space.

Side Effects
- Cardiac arrhythmia
- Hematoma
- Infection at injection site

Epidural/Combined Spinal Epidural

A catheter is placed into the dural space, and anesthesia medications are given through the catheter to block the nerve impulses from the lower spinal segments. Provides most comprehensive pain relief for delivery.

Side Effects
- Pruritus
- Hypotension
- Headache
- Fetal bradycardia
- Possible increase in length of labor
- Urinary retention

It is always important to remember it is the patient's choice. Sometimes family members will try to persuade or even want to decide the need for or the type of pain management for the patient. It is your job to advocate and support your patient's wishes, not their family members'. It is equally important to understand a patient has the right to change her mind at any time.

NITROUS OXIDE

Inhalant of 50% oxygen and 50% of nitrous oxide.

Becoming more popular in the United States; this has been used in many other developed countries for some time.

Benefits

- Self-administered so the patient stays in control of her pain management
- Allows patient to remain mobile
- No extra monitoring needed
- Short acting

Side Effects

- Vomiting
- Drowsiness
- Dizziness

Sources

American College of Obstetricians and Gynecologists' Committee on Practice Bulletins—Obstetrics. (2019). ACOG Practice Bulletin No. 209: Obstetric analgesia and anesthesia. *Obstetrics and Gynecology, 133,* e208–e225. https://doi.org/10.1097/AOG.0000000000003132

King, T., Brucker, M., Osborne, K., & Jevitt, C. M. (2018). *Varney's midwifery* (6th ed.). Jones & Bartlett Learning.

Simpson, K. R., & Creehan, P. A. (2021). *AWHONN perinatal nursing* (5th ed.). Wolters Kluwer Health.

PITOCIN

The synthetic hormone of oxytocin. It is used for labor induction and augmentation. It is also used in the immediate postpartum period to reduce PPH by causing the uterus to contract.

Fetal heart rate and uterine contractions MUST be monitored when administering Pitocin.

Side Effects
- Uterine hypertonicity
- Uterine rupture
- Abruptio placentae
- Arrhythmias
- Hypertension
- Fetal distress
- Hyperbilirubinemia of neonate
- Nausea
- Vomiting

Contraindications
- Fetal malpresentation
- Fetal distress
- MVU above 200 without progression of cervical dilatation
- Adequate contraction pattern already established
- Any contraindication for vaginal delivery
- Classical or fundal prior uterine incision
- Use with extreme caution and at a low dose for VBACs. Only to be used with women who have had a lower segment transverse uterine incision documented and in chart. (Consult the policy and procedure manual for individual institution's protocols.)

What You Need
- Pitocin
- IV pump
- Main IV fluid already infusing
- IV tubing
- Orders for administration
- Toco and EFM or IUPC and ISE in place

Administration
- If at any time infusion is being discontinued for fetal distress ordering, notify the practitioner
- Must have written order from the midwife or physician to start Pitocin with strict adherence to hospital protocol

- Must have adequate monitoring before administration to show inadequate contraction patterns and stability of FHR

Labor Induction/Augmentation

Most Common Titration
- 30 U/500 mL LR 60 mU/mL

Example
- 2 mU/min 2 mL/hr

IVPB

Start
- 1 to 2 mU/min

Increase
- 1 to 2 mU/min every 20 to 30 min PRN

Maximum Dose
- 20 mU/min

Postpartum

IV
- After delivery of placenta
  - 20 mU/L IV at 125 mL/hr
- For increased bleeding
  - 40 mU/L IV may infuse faster than 125 mL/hr depending on institutional protocol

Fast Fact

If the patient has been on Pitocin for hours and is having a PP hemorrhage, adding more Pitocin to the bag of Pitocin may not have the desired effect because her oxytocin receptors may be flooded.

IM
- 10 U IM × 1 dose after the delivery of the placenta
- If heavy bleeding continues, start IV, give 500 mL bolus of LR (if bolus is not contraindicated), and prepare to administer Methergine or Hemabate

Fast Fact

Antidote for tachysystole: Terbutaline 0.25 mg SC q 20 min PRN

Sources

American College of Obstetricians and Gynecologists' Committee on Practice Bulletins—Obstetrics. (2017). ACOG Practice Bulletin No. 183: Postpartum hemorrhage. *Ostetrics and Gynecology*, *130*(4), e168–e186. https://doi.org/10.1097/AOG.0000000000002351

Epocrates. (2020). www.epocrates.com

Simpson, K. R., & Creehan, P. A. (2021). *AWHONN perinatal nursing* (5th ed.). Wolters Kluwer Health.

RhoGAM

- Only for Rh-negative women
- Anti-D immunoglobulin (human) is given to women during their pregnancy if they are Rh negative. It stops antibody formation against the fetus if the fetus is Rh positive. It prevents newborn hemolytic disease and protects future pregnancies against alloimmunization.
- RhoGAM 300 mcg IM

Routine Administration

- 26 to 28 weeks gestational age
- Within 72 hours after delivery (if the infant is Rh positive)

Other Indications for Administration

- Maternal hx of blood transfusion
- Hx of previous newborns needing blood transfusions
- Ectopic pregnancy
- Elective or spontaneous abortion
- CVS or amniocentesis
- Fetal demise
- Second- and/or third-trimester bleeding
- Abdominal trauma

Contraindicated

- Rh-positive women
- Newborn blood type is Rh negative

Sources

American College of Obstetricians and Gynecologists' Committee on Practice Bulletins—Obstetrics. (2017). ACOG Practice Bulletin No. 181: Prevention of Rh D alloimmunization. *Obstetrics and Gynecology, 130*, e57–e70. https://doi.org/10.1097/AOG.0000000000002232

RhoGAM. (2020). www.rhogam.com

SURGICAL INSTRUMENTS

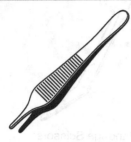

Adson Forceps

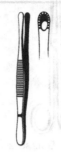

Russian Forceps

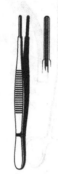

Debakey Forceps

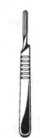

Blade/Scalpel Holder

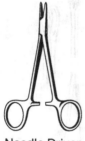

Needle Driver

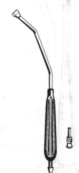

Yankauer Suction

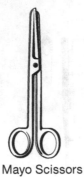

Mayo Scissors

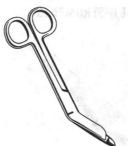

Bandage Scissors

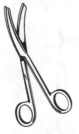

Curved Mayo

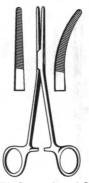

Kelly Curved and Straight

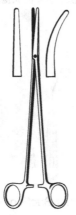

Metzenbaum Scissors

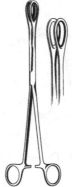

Ring Forceps/Sponge Sticks

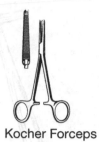

Kocher Forceps

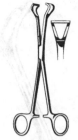

Babcock Forceps

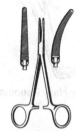

Mosquito Forceps
Curved and Straight

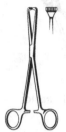

Allis Forceps

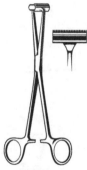

T-Clamps

Bladder Blade Retractor

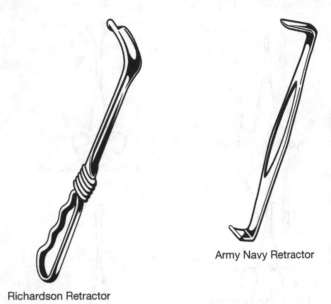

Army Navy Retractor

Richardson Retractor

Source

Groll, C. (2011). *Surgical instrument illustrations.*

VAGINAL BIRTH AFTER CESAREAN SECTION (VBAC)

Previous OR report should be in chart stating low transverse uterine incision.

Contraindications
- Previous classical incision, T-scar on uterus, fundal incision
- Previous uterine rupture
- Macrosomic fetus
- Multiple gestations
- Any contraindication to a vaginal delivery
- Less than 18 months since last C/S
- Cytotec
- The number of prior deliveries by low transverse C/S followed by a vaginal delivery is currently under debate; follow institutional guidelines

Fast Fact

Epidural and low-dose Pitocin are NOT contraindicated.

Adverse Outcomes
- Uterine rupture approximately 1%
- Failed attempt at vaginal delivery resulting in a C/S
- STAT C/S

Clinical Presentation of a Uterine Rupture
- Fetal distress
- Stabbing pain at previous C/S incision site
- Vaginal bleeding
- Fetal parts can be easily felt through abdominal wall
- Loss of station
- Unstable maternal VS
- Anticipate a STAT C/S

Sources

American College of Obstetricians and Gynecologists' Committee on Practice Bulletins—Obstetrics. (2019). ACOG Practice Bulletin No. 205: Vaginal Birth after cesarean delivery. *Obstetrics & Gynecology, 133,* e110–e127. https:// doi.org/10.1097/AOG.0000000000003078

King, T., Brucker, M., Osborne, K., & Jevitt, C. M. (2018). *Varney's midwifery* (6th ed.). Jones & Bartlett Learning.

VAGINAL DELIVERY

What You Need in the Room

- Delivery table (should be set if patient is dilated 8 cm or more and should be replaced if not used within 12 hours)
    - Most important instruments are as follows:
        - Scissors
        - Two clamps
        - Bulb suction
- Light source
- Lidocaine (Xylocaine)
- Oxytocin (Pitocin)
- Sutures
- Syringes (for lidocaine or if emergency drugs need to be administered)
- Step stool
- Cord collection kit if patient is collecting
- Mirror for mother if she wants to see the birth
- Neonatal warmer on
- Neonatal wall suction on to 100 mmHg
- Neonatal O2 on 5 to 10 L/min
- Access to the mother's antenatal blood work
- Blankets
- Oxygen
- Suction
- Diaper
- Infant hat
- Laryngoscope
- Umbilical cord clamp
- Scissors
- Thermometer
- Infant pulsometer
- Erythromycin ophthalmic ointment .5% (*administered in newborn's eyes for prophylaxis against GC/CT*)
- Vitamin K 1 kg IM 1 dose (*administered in newborns for prophylaxis of classic hemorrhagic disease*)

What to Do

- Monitor FHR
- Coach the mother on pushing and correct ineffective pushing effort
- Alert other staff that you are in a delivery
- Note the time of birth and delivery of placenta
- After delivery, place infant on mother's chest (if infant is stable)
- Assess VS

- Assess Apgar score
- Place the hat on infant
- Place a blanket on infant and mother
- Encourage breastfeeding
- If low Apgars
  - Place baby in warmer
  - Notify pediatrician
  - Stimulate baby
- After delivery of placenta, administer oxytocin (Pitocin) as ordered

How to Do a Vaginal Delivery in the Absence of a Physician or Midwife

- Apply gloves
- With one hand, apply gentle counter pressure to fetal head
- With other hand, support perineum
- Once head is out, check for umbilical cord around the neck
- If loose cord is noted, pull over head
- If tight cord is noted, use two Kelly clamps and clamp cord
- Cut between the two clamps
- Allow head to restitute in position
- Apply gentle pressure downward to deliver anterior shoulder
- Apply gentle pressure upward to deliver posterior shoulder
- Slide your posterior hand down the back as the baby delivers, and support feet as they slide over the perenium
- If not done already, clamp and cut the cord.
- Never pull on the head or use excessive pressure
- Never pull on the umbilical cord while waiting for the placenta

Source

Werner, D., Thuman, C., & Manxwell, J. (2013). *Where there is no doctor, a village health care handbook* (Rev. ed.). The Hesperian Foundation.

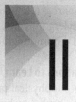

II

PROCEDURES

As a labor and delivery (L&D) nurse, you will be expected to set up for and assist with various procedures throughout a shift. Because of the nature of this ever-changing unit, any routine procedures can become emergencies very quickly. For this reason, the L&D RN must learn to anticipate possible complications and be prepared to assist both the patient and the physician or midwife.

In this section, you will find information on procedures commonly performed on L&D. The definition, indications, expected outcomes, and complications for each procedure are presented. Keep in mind that this book serves as a general guide to these procedures and does not take the place of practitioner orders or institutional protocol and guidelines. When in doubt, always ask senior nursing staff.

Medications to Know

- Carboprost (Hemabate)
- Methylergonovine (Methergine)
- $Rh_o(D)$ immunoglobulin, human (IGIM) (RhoGAM)

Abbreviations to Learn

- BPP—biophysical profile
- CPD—cephalopelvic disproportion
- d/t—due to
- fFN—fetal fibronectin
- FHR—fetal heart rate
- HTN—hypertension
- FSE or ISE—fetal/internal scalp electrode
- IUPC—intrauterine pressure catheter
- NST—nonstress test

Equipment to Locate and Become Familiar With

- Amnihook or Allis clamp
- Electronic fetal monitor (EFM)
- Fetal scalp blood sampling kit
- IUPC catheter
- Proper cable for IUPC
- Types and use of forceps
  - Simpson's forceps
  - Elliot forceps
  - Kielland forceps
  - Wrigley's forceps
  - Piper's forceps
- Ultrasound (U/S)
- Vacuum (for vacuum delivery)

AMNIOTOMY

Artificial rupture of membranes (ROM) is performed by physician or midwife to induce or expedite labor. May also be done if FHR cannot be obtained through external monitor or if FHR is nonreassuring and placement of ISE and/or IUPC is indicated.

Contraindications
- Maternal infection
- Fetus not engaged in the pelvis
- Placenta previa
- Presenting part other than the head
- Brow or face presentation

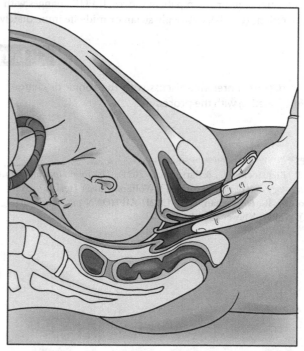

Amniotomy

Adverse Outcomes
- Cord prolapse
- Fetal injury
- Commitment to labor if the patient was not in active phase

What You Need

- Document FHR and fluid color before, during, and after the procedure
- Amnihook or Allis clamp (*should not be used in the presence of polyhydramnios*)
  - For polyhydramnios, offer ISE for a puncture of the amniotic fluid. This will allow for a trickle of amniotic fluid instead of a gush that can lead to cord prolapse.
- Sterile gloves: in appropriate sizes for the physician or midwife
- Clean white chucks or a white towel to place under the patient after rupture
- Assess and document the nature of fluid on the white chucks or towel to determine if there is meconium
- Expect continuous leaking of fluid until delivery and gushes with contractions or when patient moves. If FHR changes with decelerations (decels), notify physician or midwife immediately

Fast Fact

If the patient is preterm, discuss with the senior or charge nurse before assisting with the procedure.

Sources

Chou, B., Bienstock, J. L., & Satin, A. J. (2021). *The John Hopkins manual of gynecology and obstetrics* (6th ed.). Wolters Kluwer Health.

Simpson, K. R., & Creehan, P. A. (2021) *AWHONN perinatal nursing* (5th ed.). Wolters Kluwer Health.

AMNIOINFUSION

The process of adding fluid into the uterus through intrauterine catheter. To be done only by a physician or midwife.

Indications
- Variable decelerations
- Oligohydramnios

Contraindications
- Malpresentation
- Maternal infection
- Vaginal bleeding of unknown origin
- Placenta previa
- Placental abruption
- Ominous fetal heart tracing
- Umbilical cord prolapse

What You Need
- Sterile gloves
- IUPC catheter (if not already placed)
- IV pump and tubing
- Proper cable for IUPC
- IV fluid (normal saline)

On Pump
- Bolus 500 mL of fluid over 30 min
- Continuous drip of 100 to 250 mL/hr
- *Bolus and continuous rates should be followed as ordered; if in doubt of the proper institutional rates, check the policy and procedure manual*

Guidelines for amniotomy should be followed if the membranes are intact before procedure.

Fast Fact

Always check to be sure that there is an adequate amount of fluid outflow. If no fluid outflow is noted, notify the practitioner immediately and stop infusion.

Sources

King, T., Brucker, M., Osborne, K., & Jevitt, C. M. (2018). *Varney's midwifery* (6th ed.). Jones and Bartlett.

Chou, B., Bienstock J. L., & Satin, A. J. (2021). *The John Hopkins manual of gynecology and obstetrics* (6th ed.). Wolters Kluwer Health.

Simpson, K. R., & Creehan, P. A. (2021). *AWHONN perinatal nursing* (5th ed.). Wolters Kluwer Health.

BIOPHYSICAL PROFILE (BPP)

U/S surveillance used to assess the fetal breathing, movements, tone (all must be observed within 30 minutes of each other), and amniotic fluid volume. A nonstress test may not be ordered if U/S assessment is completely normal. To score, each test is rated as 2 (*normal*) or 0 (*abnormal*).

Interpretation of Scoring

- 8 to 10—reassuring
- 6—equivocal test; should be repeated in 24 hours if the patient has not delivered or been induced
- 4 or less—abnormal; the patient most likely will be admitted and delivered; clinical management will depend on gestational age and full clinical picture

Indications

- Postdates
- Intrauterine growth restriction (IUGR)
- Gestational diabetes/type 1 diabetes
- Multiple gestations
- Chronic or pregnancy-induced hypertension
- Hx of fetal demise
- Decreased fetal movement
- Oligohydramnios
- High-risk pregnancy due to maternal health conditions
- Patient may be assessed as often as 2×/wk, beginning at 32 weeks; clinical context will predict when to initiate BPP and the frequency
- Maternal obesity—surveillance begins after 36 weeks

Sources

American College of Obstetricians and Gynecologists. (2014). ACOG Practice Bulletin No. 145: Antepartum fetal surveillance. *Obstetrics & Gynecology, 124*, 182–192. https://doi.org/10.1097/01.AOG.0000451759.90082.7b.

Chou, B., Bienstock, J. L., & Satin, A. J. (2021). *The John Hopkins manual of gynecology and obstetrics* (6th ed.). Wolters Kluwer Health.

King, T., Brucker, M., Osborne, K., & Jevitt, C. M. (2018) *Varney's midwifery* (6th ed.). Jones and Bartlett.

EXTERNAL CEPHALIC VERSION

The process in which a breech or transverse fetus is turned into the cephalic position through the abdominal wall. Should only be performed on patients who are 37 weeks gestation or more.

Contraindications
- Fetal distress
- Low amniotic fluid
- Placenta previa
- Fetal anomalies
- HTN (uncontrolled or pregnancy induced)
- Uterine malformation
- Vaginal delivery contraindicated

Risks
- Fetal distress/demise
- Uterine rupture
- Placental abruption
- Labor
- Amniotic fluid embolism
- STAT C/S

What You Need
- First obtain a reactive NST, well documented
- Establish IV access
- Type and screen, complete blood count (CBC)
- If patient is Rh negative, give RhoGAM and document that the patient has received it
- Blood bank with 2 units on standby
- U/S machine in room
- Gel for mother's abdomen

Orders to Be Expected
- IV fluids
- Tocolytics
- Pain management for mother
- RhoGAM 300 mcg IM in Rh-negative women after procedure
- NST after procedure

Fast Fact

This procedure should ONLY be done if there is an OR with personnel on standby if the need for an STAT C/S occurs.

Sources

American College of Obstetricians and Gynecologists. (2020). ACOG Practice Bulletin No. 221: External cephalic version. *Obstetrics & Gynecology, 135*, e203–e212. https://doi.org/10.1097/AOG.0000000000003837

Cunningham, G., & Leveno, K. J. (2018). *Williams obstetrics* (25th ed.). McGraw-Hill.

FETAL FIBRONECTIN (fFN)

Vaginal swab used to predict the likelihood a patient will go into labor within the next 2 weeks. Should be done between 24 and 35 weeks and every 2 weeks as indicated. Must be done before vaginal exam, vaginal cultures, or vaginal U/S. Sample should be taken from the posterior fornix of the vagina rotating the swab gently for 10 seconds. For symptomatic patients 24 to 35 weeks, asymptotic patients 22 to 31 weeks.

Indications
- History of preterm delivery
- Symptoms of preterm labor

What You Need
- Speculum
- Sterile gloves
- Adequate light source
- fFN swab

Conditions Resulting in Test Inaccuracy
- ROM
- Bleeding present
- Patient has had sex or vaginal exam within 24 hours of the test (if results are negative this can be accurate; if test is positive repeat in 24 hours)
- Medication or lubrication present
- Cervix is dilated greater than 3 cm
- Patient has vaginal infection
- Malpresentation of placenta
- Placental abruption

Interpretation of Results
- Negative = 99% that patient will not deliver within 7 to 10 days
- Positive = 87% that patient will deliver within 7 days

Fast Fact

Use water to help glide the speculum into the vagina instead of vaginal gel.

Sources
fFNTest.com. (2020). Fetal Fibronectin In-Service (Webinar). https://hologiced .com/training/fetal-fibronectin-in-service-webinar

Chou, B., Bienstock, J. L., & Satin, A. J. (2021) *The John Hopkins manual of gynecology and obstetrics* (6th ed.). Wolters Kluwer Health.

Lab Tests Online. (2020). https://labtestsonline.org/tests/fetal-fibronectin-ffn

NONSTRESS TEST (NST)

Evaluation of fetal well-being using EFM to monitor FHR.

Indications

- Decreased fetal movement
- Postdates
- Maternal history of gestational diabetes mellitus (GDM) or diabetes mellitus type 1 or 2
- Maternal HTN
- Known fetal anomalies
- IUGR
- Twins
- Abnormal amniotic fluid index
- Poor maternal weight gain
- Maternal history of intrauterine fetal demise (IUFD)

What You Need

- Toco
- EFM
- Gel for monitor
- Bands to keep monitor in place

Reactive NST

- Fetal heart baseline should be between 110 and 160 bpm
- Less than 32 weeks, two or more accelerations rising 10 bpm above baseline for 10 seconds each
- Greater than 32 weeks, two or more accelerations rising 15 bpm above baseline for 15 seconds each

Nonreactive NST

Failure to meet preceding criteria within a 40-minute time frame.

Sources

American College of Obstetricians and Gynecologists. (2014). ACOG Practice Bulletin No. 145: Antepartum fetal surveillance. *Obstetrics & Gynecology*, *124*, 182–192. https://doi.org/10.1097/01.AOG.0000451759.90082.7b

King, T., Brucker, M., Osborne, K., & Jevitt, C. M. (2018). *Varney's midwifery* (6th ed.). Jones and Bartlett.

OPERATIVE VAGINAL DELIVERY

The use of either forceps or vacuum to assist with a vaginal delivery.

Indications
- Maternal exhaustion
- Inadequate/prolonged pushing
- Fetal distress
- Cardiac delivery

Complications
- Maternal lacerations: cervical, vaginal, and possible damage to anal sphincter
- Episiotomy
- Postpartum hemorrhage
- Trauma to urethra and/or bladder
- Newborn lacerations
- Skull fracture
- Nerve damage: maternal and fetal
- Intracranial bleed

Requirements
- Fully dilated
- Fetal head engaged in pelvis
- Maternal bladder empty
- No suspicion of CPD
- Gestational age greater than 36 weeks

What to Do
- Notify pediatrician
- Set up room for vaginal delivery
- Place forceps or vacuum on delivery table in a sterile manner
- Have methylergonovine (Methergine) and carboprost (Hemabate) available
- Place step stool in room
- Request a more senior nurse to assist with delivery

Types of Forceps
- Simpson's forceps: most common
- Elliot forceps: should only be used in multiparous women
- Kielland forceps: used for rotating the baby
- Wrigley's forceps: used in low or outlet delivery
- Piper's forceps: used in breech deliveries

Criteria of Forceps
- Outlet forceps: fetal scalp remains visible when the mother is not pushing

- Low forceps: fetal station is +2 or below
- Midforceps: fetal head engaged but above +2 station

Vacuum Delivery

- General rule is maximum of three pulls (follow your institution's guidelines)
- Popoffs indicate too much force without progression of fetal head descent
  - They should not be accepted as routine, and a maximum of three popoffs should indicate need for other methods of delivery.
- No more than 600 mmHg of pressure should be used
- Maximum vacuum time from placement until detachment or delivery should not exceed 30 minutes

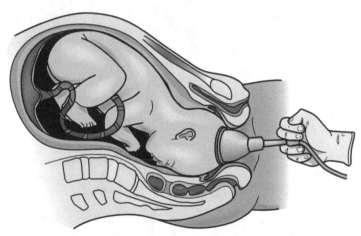

Vacuum Delivery

Sources

Cunningham, G., & Leveno. K. J. (2018). *Williams obstetrics* (25th ed.). McGraw-Hill.

Simpson, K. R., & Creehan, P. A. (2021). *AWHONN perinatal nursing* (5th ed.). Wolters Kulwer Health.

American College of Obstetricians and Gynecologists. (2020). ACOG Practice Bulletin No. 219: Operative vaginal birth. *Obstetrics & Gynecology, 135*, e149–159. https://doi.org/10.1097/AOG.0000000000003764

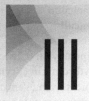

EMERGENCIES

As labor and delivery (L&D) is a fast-paced unit, many hospitals consider it an ICU and limit the number of patients assigned per RN to two. This is because complications can (and do) arise without notice. On "good days," the majority of your patients will be healthy with a normal progression of labor and delivery of a healthy beautiful newborn. On "other days," your patients might be acutely ill with complications related or unrelated to the pregnancy.

These are the patients whom you must observe carefully for subtle changes in either the mother or the baby and know how to respond immediately when necessary to those changes. You are the first line of care for your patient. It is your responsibility to be informed of potential complications and, when related changes occur, to tell the physician or midwife about these changes immediately.

In this section, you will find the more common complications and emergencies that you will encounter in L&D. This is an important section. Read it over and over until you feel totally familiar with the content so that you can act competently and appropriately when a complication arises. During an actual emergency, there is little time to look at a reference book.

Medications to Know

- Ampicillin
- Penicillin
- Gentamicin
- Clindamycin (Cleocin)
- Erythromycin (Erythrocin)
- Vancomycin (Vancocin)
- Magnesium sulphate
- Calcium gluconate
- Labetalol (Trandate)
- Hydralazine
- Betamethasone (Celestone)
- Dexamethasone
- Lorazepam (Ativan)
- Oxytocin (Pitocin)
- Methylergonovine (Methergine)
- Carboprost (Hemabate)
- Misoprostol (Cytotec)
- Indomethacin (Indocin)
- Nifedipine (Procardia)
- Terbutaline
- Dinoprostone (Cervidil, Prepidil)

Abbreviations to Learn

- C/S—cesarean section
- DIC—disseminated intracoagulopathy
- HELLP—hemolysis elevated liver enzymes low platelet count
- PPH—postpartum haemorrhage
- PPROM—preterm premature rupture of membranes
- U/S—ultrasound

Equipment to Locate and to Become Familiar With

- Neonate crash cart

ABRUPTIO PLACENTAE

Separation of placenta from uterine wall before delivery.

Risk Factors
- Scar on uterus (prior myomectomy or C/S)
- Blunt abdominal trauma
- Hx of previous abruptio placentae
- Hypertension (HTN)
- Multiparity
- PPROM
- Cocaine use
- Advanced maternal age (AMA)
- Smoking
- Chorioamnionitis

Clinical Presentation
- Acute localized uterine pain
- Frank bleeding
- Occult bleeding (need U/S to determine)
- Back pain
- Fetal distress
- Tetanic contractions—no resting tone

Whom to Call
- GET HELP IMMEDIATELY
- Physician/midwife to bedside immediately
- Senior nursing staff
- Alert on-call pediatrician
- Rapid response team/code team

What to Do
- Establish continuous fetal heart rate (FHR)
- Anticipate possible need for internal fetal monitoring
- IV access with 18G needle (if not already done)
- Establish a second line with 18G for blood administration (if needed)
- Monitor maternal vital signs (VS)
- Call blood bank and have 2 units of packed RBC crossmatched
- Anticipate probable C/S (not always indicated)
- Obtain portable U/S in room

Labs
- Complete blood count (CBC)
- Type and screen

- Type and crossmatch for 2 units
- PT/PTT
- Fibrinogen
- Fibrin split products
- Toxicology

Fast Facts

- Patients with abruption may have precipitous deliveries.
- Anticipate possible PPH or DIC.

Sources

Cunningham, G., & Leveno, K. J. (2018). *Williams obstetrics* (25th ed.). McGraw-Hill.

Hurt, K. J., Guile, M. W., Bienstock, J. L., Fox, H. E., & Wallach, E. E. (2020). *The Johns Hopkins manual of gynecology and obstetrics* (6th ed.). Lippincott Williams & Wilkins.

Mei, Y., & Lin, Y. (2018). Clinical significance of primary symptoms in women with placental abruption. *The Journal of Maternal-Fetal and Neonatal Medicine, 18*, 2446–2449. https://doi.org/10.1080/14767058.20 17.1344830

Simpson, K. R., Creehan, P. A., O'Brien-Abel, N., Roth, C., & Rohan, A. J. (2020). *Perinatal nursing* (5th ed.). Lippincott Williams & Wilkins.

AMNIOTIC FLUID EMBOLISM

It is a rare complication in which amniotic fluid or fetal debris crosses the placenta into maternal circulation. It can occur during labor or postpartum.

Risk Factors
- Induction of labor
- Operative delivery
- Mutiparity
- Advanced maternal age
- Placenta previa
- Abdominal trauma
- Diabetes
- Cervical lacerations
- Placenta abruption
- Uterine rupture

Clinical Presentation
- Dyspnea
- Cyanosis
- Fetal distress (if undelivered)
- Maternal hypotension
- Maternal cardiac arrest

Whom to Call
- GET HELP IMMEDIATELY
- Call covering physician STAT if midwife is managing patient
- Anesthesia STAT
- All senior nursing staff available to help

What to Do
- Give O2 through facemask
- Call blood bank for
    - Two units of packed RBC crossed and matched brought STAT
    - Fresh frozen plasma STAT
- Access another IV site with 18G needle
- Anticipate STAT C/S and full maternal code (prep patient for C/S and have the crash cart ready)

Labs
- Type and screen (if admission labs not obtained)
- Arterial blood gases
- Serum electrolytes
- Comprehensive metabolic panel (CMP)
- Coagulation profile

- CBC
- Type and crossmatch for 2 units

Fast Fact

If the patient survives delivery, there is a high risk for DIC.

Sources

Cunningham, G., & Leveno, K. J. (2018). *Williams obstetrics* (25th ed.). McGraw-Hill.

Clark, S. L. (2018). Managing obstetric emergencies: Anaphylactoid syndrome of pregnancy (aka AFE): Ob/gyns must be ready to move quickly when a patient exhibits the sudden and unexpected signs of anaphylactoid syndrome (ASP). *Contemporary OB/GYN, 63*(7).

McBride, A. M. (2018). Clinical presentation and treatment of amniotic fluid embolism. *AACN Advanced Critical Care, 29*(3), 336–342. https://doi.org/10.4037/aacnacc2018419

Hurt, K. J., Guile, M. W., Bienstock, J. L., Fox, H. E., & Wallach, E. E. (2020). *The Johns Hopkins manual of gynecology and obstetrics* (6th ed.). Lippincott Williams & Wilkins.

BLEEDING IN PREGNANCY

Causes in second and third trimester

Painful	Painless
Labor term or preterm	Placenta previa
Placenta abruption	Loss of mucous plug
Uterine rupture	Polyp on cervix (mostly seen after intercourse)
Trauma	

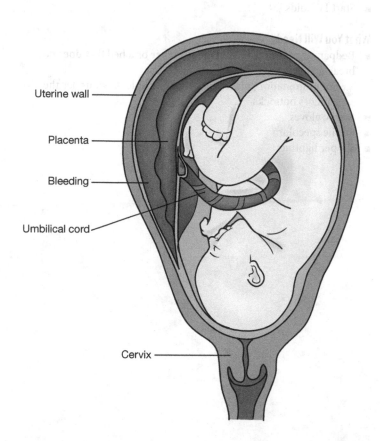

Uterine wall

Placenta

Bleeding

Umbilical cord

Cervix

Abruption

Never do a vaginal exam if the cause of bleeding is unknown. Notify the practitioner immediately.

What to Do
- Call practitioner on call
- Call senior nursing staff
- Maternal VS
- Monitor fetus with electronic fetal monitoring (EFM) and Toco
- Start IV fluids LR

What You Will Need
- Bedpan (if patient is in a triage stretcher or a bed that does not break apart)
  - For examination, place the bedpan upside down under the patient's buttocks
- Sterile gloves
- Sterile speculum
- Proper lighting

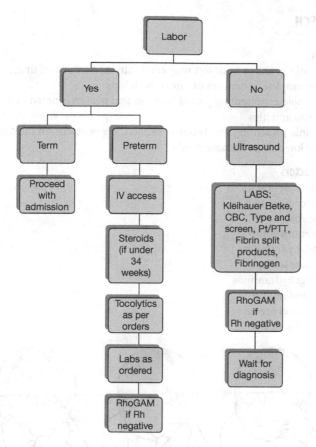

Bleeding in Pregnancy

Sources

Cunningham, G., & Leveno, K. J. (2018). *Williams obstetrics* (25th ed.).
  McGraw-Hill.

Hurt, K. J., Guile, M. W., Bienstock, J. L., Fox, H. E., & Wallach, E. E.
  (2020). *The Johns Hopkins manual of gynecology and obstetrics* (6th ed.).
  Lippincott Williams & Wilkins.

BREECH

Types
- Footling: one or both feet may enter into the birth canal first, (incomplete) extension of one or both hips
- Complete: presenting part is buttocks and flexion is noted in both knees and hips
- Frank: presenting part is buttocks and there is extension through the knees (feet are near head)

Risk Factors
- Multiple gestations
- Bicornuate uterus
- Fibroids
- Preterm labor
- Polyhydramnios
- Macrosomia
- Oligohydramnios
- Grand multip
- Placenta previa
- Fetal issues

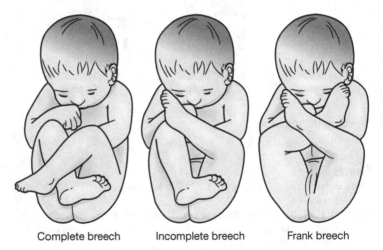

Complete breech   Incomplete breech   Frank breech

Adverse Effects
- Cord prolapse
- Fetal injury
- Fetal asphyxia
- Mortality
- Head entrapment (cervix may not be fully dilated)

What to Do
- Delivery eminent
  - Call for help; notify pediatrician STAT
  - Monitor fetus
  - If cord prolapse noted, put mother in Trendelenburg and try to relieve pressure on umbilical cord using a vaginal hand (*see* Umbilical cord prolapse)
- Delivery not imminent
  - Monitor fetus
  - Call the on-call practitioner STAT
- Prep for C/S

What You Need for a Vaginal Breech Delivery
- Delivery tray (at least a pair of sterile scissors and lidocaine)
- For leverage, bring the mother to edge of bed or break the bed, if time
- Warm towel (practitioner will need during delivery to apply around neonate's body)
- IV access: 18G needle
- Neonate crash cart
- Pediatrician in room

Sources
Cunningham, G., & Leveno, K. J. (2018). *Williams obstetrics* (25th ed.). McGraw-Hill.

Hurt, K. J, Guile, M. W., Bienstock, J. L., Fox, H. E., & Wallach, E. E. (2020). *The Johns Hopkins manual of gynecology and obstetrics* (6th ed.). Lippincott Williams & Wilkins.

King, T. L., Brucker, M. C., Osborne, K., & Jevitt, C. M. (2019). *Varney's midwifery* (6th ed.). Jones & Bartlett Learning.

CHORIOAMNIONITIS

Infection of placenta, chorion, and amnion

Risk Factors

- Prolonged labor
- Primip's
- PROM/PPROM/prolonged rupture of membranes
- Serial vaginal exams
- Intrauterine pressure catheter (IUPC)/internal scalp electrode (ISE)
- Vaginal infections (i.e., bacterial vaginosis [BV] or group B *Streptococcus* [GBS])

Clinical Presentation

Maternal	Fetal
Temp of 38°C	Tachycardia
Tachycardia	Amniotic fluid has foul odor
Increased white blood cell (WBC) count	Low Apgars
Tender abdomen	Acidosis
Labor dystocia	
Foul-smelling vaginal discharge	

What to Expect

- Induction of labor
- Augmentation to hasten labor
- VS ordered q hour
- Antibiotic therapy (note whether the patient has allergies)
- Hydration with IV fluids
- If no PCN allergy
  - Ampicillin 2 g IVPB q 6 hr until delivery with gentamicin 2 mg/kg IVPB to load then 1.5 mg/kg IVPB q 8 hr until delivery.
  - Ampicillin 2 g intravenous piggyback (IVPB) × 1 dose, then 1 g 4 hr
  - Gentamicin 120 mg IVPB × 1 dose, then 80 mg IVPB q 8 hr
- If PCN allergy
  - Cefazolin 1 g IVPB q 8 hr for ampicillin until delivery
  - Clindamycin (Cleocin) 900 mg IVPB q 8 hr
  - Erythromycin (Erythrocin) 1 g IVPB q 6 hr
  - Vancomycin (Vancocin) 500 mg IVPB q 6 hr

Fast Facts

The pediatrician should be notified and present at the delivery. Each hospital may have a policy for managing the infant. The placenta may be sent to pathology.

Sources

Conde-Agudelo, A., Romero, R., JungJung, E., & Sanchez, A. J. G. (2020). Management of clinical chorioamnionitis: An evidence-based approach. *American Journal of Obstetrics and Gynecology, 223*(6), 848–869. https://doi.org/10.1016/j.ajog.2020.09.044

Hurt, K. J, Guile, M. W., Bienstock, J. L., Fox, H. E., & Wallach, E. E. (2020). *The Johns Hopkins manual of gynecology and obstetrics* (6th ed.). Lippincott Williams & Wilkins.

King, T. L., Brucker, M. C., Osborne, K., & Jevitt, C. M. (2019). *Varney's midwifery* (6th ed.). Jones & Bartlett Learning.

HYPERTENSION/HYPERTENSIVE DISORDERS IN PREGNANCY

Preeclampsia

Develops after 20 weeks gestation and patient is usually symptomatic with proteinuria, headache, visual disturbances, N/V, rapid weight gain, decreased urine output, and epigastric pain. Cause is unknown.

Diagnosis

Mild Preeclampsia

■ 140 systolic or 90 diastolic or higher (at least 6 hours apart) after 20 weeks gestational diabetes age (GA) with no hx of HTN

Proteinuria greater than .3 g/d in 24-hour urine or 1+ urine protein dipstick

Severe Preeclampsia

■ 160 mmHg systolic and 110 mmHg diastolic
■ Proteinuria 5 g or more in results of 24-hour urine collection/ ≥3+ urine protein dipstick
■ Oliguria less than 500 mL in 24-hour urine results
■ Pulmonary edema/crackles
■ Epigastric pain

Risk Factors

■ Primip
■ Multiple gestations
■ Diabetes
■ Teen pregnancy
■ Advanced maternal age
■ Smoker
■ Obesity
■ Previous history of preeclampsia
■ Chronic hypertension
■ Reproductive conception

Complications

■ Seizure
■ HELLP syndrome
■ Intrauterine growth restriction (IUGR)
■ Abruptio placentae

Labs

- CBC
- Liver function panel
- Kidney function panel
- PT/PTT
- Fibrinogen
- Urine dipstick/urinalysis
- 24-hour urine protein collection

Lab Interpretation

- Elevated
  - LDH
  - Serum creatinine
  - Uric acid greater than 6 mg
  - AST/ALT
  - Proteinuria

Medications (Administer as Ordered)

Seizure Prevention

Recommend to review Magnesium Protocol for Seizure Prevention

- Magnesium sulfate (MgSO4) loading dose 4 to 6 g IV, then 2 to 4 g IV/hr
- If no IV access, give 5 g magnesium sulfate (50% solution) IM in each buttock (10 g total), with a maintenance dose of 5 g in alternating buttocks every 4 hr
  - Serum mg level should be drawn q 6 hr. Levels should be between 6 and 8 mg/dL (Johns Hopkins states a therapeutic range of 4–6)
    - Mg levels 8 to 10 mg/dL decrease deep tendon reflexes
  - Greater than >12 ECG changes and cardiac arrythmias 15 mg/dL cardiac arrest
  - Monitor I&Os and IV fluid needs to be managed, no more than 125 mL/hr of total if IV fluids is infusing
  - Fluid volume limit of 3,000 mL intake per 24 hr while on magnesium

Fast Facts

Antidote (hypermagnesemia): Calcium gluconate 1 g IV over 3 min; Rapid infusion can result in cardiac arrest. **Should be in room if MgSO4 is infusing**. RN does not need to be in the room for full infusion time.

HTN Control
- Labetalol (Trandate) 20 mg IV push, then escalating 10-min intervals of 20, 40, 80, 80, 80 mg for max 300 mg/24 hr
- Hydralazine 5 mg IV bolus q 20 min to maximum of 20 mg PRN

Steroids for Fetal Lung Maturity If Preterm
- Betamethasone (Celestone) 12 mg IM q 24 hr × 2
- Dexamethasone 6 mg IM q 12 hr × 4

HELLP Syndrome
- Acronym stands for
  - **H**—hemolysis
  - **EL**—elevated liver enzymes
  - **LP**—low platelet count
- Risk factors, symptoms, and treatment are similar to preeclampsia.

Labs
- CBC
- Liver function panel
- Kidney function panel
- PT/PTT
- Fibrinogen
- Urine dipstick/urinalysis
- 24-hour urine protein collection

Lab Interpretation
- Hemolysis
- Increased liver enzymes
- Low platelets

Eclampsia
- Preceded by preeclampsia, but patient has suffered from seizure activity and/or coma.

Management of a Seizure
Whom to Call
- GET HELP IMMEDIATELY
- Notify attending physician STAT
- Notify anesthesia STAT
- All senior nursing staff available to help
- Notify pediatrician: should be on standby for STAT C/S

What to Do
- Secure the area so that the patient is safe while having seizure
- ABCs
- Give O2 through a face mask

- Anticipate fetal bradycardia
- Access another IV site with 18G needle
- Anticipate STAT C/S once FHR has stabilized or has been bradycardic for longer than 10 minutes

Medications (Administer as Ordered)
- Magnesium sulfate (MgSO4) 4–6 g IV bolus
  - If seizure occurs during or after loading dose, bolus another 2 g
- If seizure activity persists, lorazepam (Ativan) .1 mg/kg IV or phenytoin (Dilantin) 1,000–1,250-mg loading dose (most likely administered by anesthesia)

Sources

American College of Obstetricians and Gynecologists. (2001). Chronic hypertension in pregnancy (Practice Bulletin No. 29). In *2008 Compendium of Selected Publications* (pp. 686–694). Washington, D.C.: Author.

American College of Obstetricians and Gynecologists. (2002). Diagnosis and management of preeclampsia and eclampsia (Practice Bulletin No. 33). In *2008 Compendium of Selected Publications* (pp. 717–725). Washington, D.C.: Author.

American College of Obstetricians and Gynecologists. (2020). ACOG Practice Bulletin No. 222: Gestational hypertension and preeclampsia. *Obstetrics and Gynecology, 135*(6), 1492–1495. https://doi.org/10.1097/AOG.0000000000003891

Booker, W. A. (2020). Hypertensive disorders of pregnancy. *Clinics in Perinatology, 47*(4), 817–833. https://doi.org/10.1016/j.clp.2020.08.011

Brown, M. A., Magee, L. A., Kenny, L. C., Karumanchi, A., McCarthy, F. P., Saito, S., Hall, D. R., Warren, C. E., Adoyi, G., & Ishaku, S. (2018). Hypertensive disorders of pregnancy. *Hypertension, 72*(1), 24–43. https://doi.org/10.1161/HYPERTENSIONAHA.117.10803

Hurt, K. J., Guile, M. W., Bienstock, J. L., Fox, H. E., & Wallach, E. E. (2020). *The Johns Hopkins manual of gynecology and obstetrics* (6th ed.). Lippincott Williams & Wilkins.

MECONIUM

Meconium is the first bowel movement of the fetus or newborn. Not uncommon at term. Also known as Mec.

Risk Factors
- Term or postterm
- Fetal distress
- Long labor
- Maternal hypertension
- Gestational diabetes

Clinical Presentation
- Can only be noted after ROM
- Note consistency (light, moderate, thick, heavy)
- Because it can be associated with fetal distress, note the FHR and tracing often throughout the labor

Whom to Call
- Notify midwife or physician
- Notify pediatrician—they should be present at delivery

Adverse Outcome
- Meconium aspiration syndrome—when the newborn breathes in a mix of meconium and amniotic fluid. This can make breathing very difficult or impossible for the newborn.

What to Do
- Have a second nurse at the delivery to help
- Hand newborn immediately to awaiting pediatrician
- Have the room properly stocked and prepared for neonate resuscitation

What You Need
- Neonatal O2 on 5 to 10 L/min
- Stethoscope
- Wall suction with tubing set to 100 mmHg
- Meconium aspirator
- Laryngoscope
- Appropriate-sized endotracheal tubes

Fast Fact

It was common practice until only a few years ago to do an amnioinfusion during labor for meconium. Research shows that there is no beneficial evidence for an amnioinfusion or suctioning a newborn on the perineum before delivery of the shoulders.

Sources

Chiruvolu, A., Miklis, K. K., Chen, E., Petrey, B., & Desai, S. (2018). Delivery room management of meconium-stained newborns and respiratory support. *Pediatrics, 142*(6), 1485. https://doi.org/10.1542/peds.2018-1485

Kalra, V. K., Lee, H., Sie, L., Ratnasiri, A. W., Underwood, M. A., & Lakshminrusimha, S. (2020). Change in neonatal resuscitation guidelines and trends in incidence of meconium aspiration syndrome in California. *Journal of Perinatology, 40*, 46–55. https://doi.org/10.1038/s41372-019-0529-0

King, T. L., Brucker, M. C., Osborne, K., & Jevitt, C. M. (2019). *Varney's midwifery* (6th ed.). Jones & Bartlett Learning.

Simpson, K. R., Creehan, P. A., O'Brien-Abel, N., Roth, C., & Rohan, A. J. (2020). *Perinatal nursing* (5th ed.). Lippincott Williams & Wilkins.

PLACENTAL ABNORMALITIES

Placenta Previa

As the uterus grows, the placenta moves and previas may resolve by time of delivery. U/S is needed to rule out previous previa at term if not already done.

Definitions

- Low lying: the placenta is close to the edge of the os
- Marginal: the placenta has reached the edge of the os
- Partial: the placenta is covering some of the os
- Complete: the placenta is completely covering the os
- Vasa previa: cord insertion is through membranes instead of placenta

Risk Factors

- Multiparity
- Prior uterine surgery
- Advanced maternal age
- Smoking
- Abnormality of uterus

Fast Fact

Sterile vaginal exam (SVE) and vaginal delivery are contraindicated.

Whom to Call

- GET HELP IMMEDIATELY
- Call covering physician STAT if midwife is managing patient
- Notify anesthesia STAT
- Notify pediatrician STAT
- Call all senior nursing staff available to help

What to Do

- DO NOT DO A VAGINAL EXAM
- Prepare for a STAT C/S
  - Start IV LR 18G
  - Admission labs
  - Call the blood bank for 2 units crossed and matched
  - Bicitra (if time)
  - Foley catheter

- Consent
- ID bands
- Monitor FHR

Placenta Accreta/Increta/Percreta

May be diagnosed after delivery of neonate when the placenta fails to deliver as expected. The patient may be taken to the OR for post-delivery dilatation and curettage (D&C) or possible hysterectomy if bleeding cannot be controlled.

Definitions

- Accreta: placenta attaches to myometrium without the decidua basalis
- Increta: attaches into the myometrium
- Percreta: placenta permeates through the myometrium and may affect the bladder and/or bowel

What to Expect

- Possible C/S hysterectomy

Sources

Cunningham, G., & Leveno, K. J. (2018). *Williams obstetrics* (25th ed.). McGraw-Hill.

Hurt, K. J., Guile, M. W., Bienstock, J. L., Fox, H. E., & Wallach, E. E. (2020). *The Johns Hopkins manual of gynecology and obstetrics* (6th ed.). Lippincott Williams & Wilkins.

Simpson, K. R., Creehan, P. A., O'Brien-Abel, N., Roth, C., & Rohan, A. J. (2020). *Perinatal nursing* (5th ed.). Lippincott Williams & Wilkins.

POSTPARTUM HEMORRHAGE

Greater than 500 mL blood loss for a vaginal delivery and 1,000 mL blood loss after cesarean delivery. Hemodynamic instability may occur with less blood loss if patient is anemic. Can also be diagnosed with a 10% drop of hematocrit (HCT).

Risk Factors

- Anemia
- Overdistended uterus
- Prolonged Pitocin induction/augmentation
- Infection
- Retained placenta
- Prolonged labor
- Fibroids
- Lacerations during delivery
- Operative delivery
- Maternal coagulation deficiencies

What to Do

- GET HELP IMMEDIATELY
- Start IV 18G (if not previously done)
- Start second 18G IV for blood products
- Give IV fluid resuscitation
- Empty bladder with catheter
- Monitor maternal VS (tachycardia early sign and tachycardia with hypotension a late sign)
- Give O2 through nonrebreather face mask
- Administration of Methergine/Hemabate/Pitocin/Cytotec as ordered
- Call blood bank: 2 units crossed and matched STAT
- Anticipate possible transfer to the OR for D&C or hysterectomy if bleeding is unable to be controlled
- Recommend to also do balloon tamponade
- Weigh all pads and linens for accuracy 1 g = 1 mL blood loss

Medications (Administer as Ordered)

- Oxytocin (Pitocin): 10 IU/mL IM or 40 U IV—should have in room at every delivery
- Methylergonovine (Methergine): .2 mg IM q 2 to 4 hr—do not give to HTN/preeclamptic patients/Reynaud's/smoker
    - SHOULD BE KEPT IN REFRIGERATOR
- Carboprost (Hemabate) 250 mcg IM q 15 to 90 min max 8 doses—may cause maternal N/V/D
- Do not give with hx of asthma

- Misoprostol (Cytotec) 800 to 1,000 mcg rectal—may cause maternal fever and diarrhea in the breastfeeding newborn
- Dinoprostone (Cervidil, Prepidil) 20 mg PR/PV q 2 hr

Sources

Borovac-Pinheiro, A., Pacagnella, R. C., Cecatti, J. G., Miller, S., El Ayadi, A. M., Souza, J. P., Durocher, J., Blumenthal, P. D., & Winikoff, B. (2018). Postpartum hemorrhage: New insights for definition and diagnosis. *American Journal of Obstetrics and Gynecology, 219*(2), 162–168. https://doi.org/10.1016/j.ajog.2018.04.013

King, T. L., Brucker, M. C., Osborne, K., & Jevitt, C. M. (2019). *Varney's midwifery* (6th ed.). Jones & Bartlett Learning.

PREMATURITY

Preterm L&D

Between weeks 20 and 37 of gestational age with regular uterine contractions (UCX) and cervical dilatation or rupture of membranes (ROM).

Risk Factors

- Multiple gestations
- Polyhydramnios
- Previous PTL or PTL delivery
- Placenta previa/abruption
- Maternal age <18 and >40
- Infection
- No prenatal care
- Smoking
- Substance abuse

What to Do

- Monitor FHR and UCX patterns
- Start IV and hydrate
- Maternal VS
- Admission labs
- Evaluation of PROM
- Prepare supplies for sterile speculum exam

What to Expect

- Anticipate sterile speculum exam
- U/S/cervical length
- Fetal fibronectin (fFN; 24–34 weeks gestation)
- Continuous fetal monitoring
- Admission
- Anticipate delivery more than 34 weeks and PPROM

Labs

- CBC
- Urinalysis
- Urine culture and sensitivity (obtained through straight catheter)
- Vaginal cultures
- Ffn

Medications (Administer as Ordered)

- Corticosteroids—for fetal lung maturity (between 24–34 weeks)
  - Betamethasone (Celestone) 12 mg IM q 24 hr × 2 doses

- Dexamethasone 6 mg IM q 12 hr × 4 doses
- Tocolytics—to try to stop labor
  - Indomethacin (Indocin) 50 to 100 mg PO or per rectum at first dose, then 25 to 50 mg PO q 4 to 6 hr × 72 hr (not to exceed 72 hr). Do not give if >32 weeks gestation due to premature closure of the fetus ductus arteriosus.
    - Do not give if oligohydramnios
  - Nifedipine (Procardia) 10 to 20 mg PO q 6 hr
  - Terbutaline .25 mg SQ q 20 to 30 min PRN
    - May cause maternal tachycardia
    - Do not give to diabetics; will increase blood sugars
  - Magnesium sulfate for infant neuroprotection 4 g bolus followed by either 1 g/hr × 24 hr or 2 g hr × 12 hr

Definitions of gestational age and timing for delivery indications

Late preterm	34 0/7–36 6/7 weeks
Early term	37 0/7–38 6/7 weeks
Term	39 0/7–40 6/7 weeks
Late term	41 0/7–41 6/7 weeks
Postterm	42 weeks and beyond

All women experiencing normal pregnancies should not be induced or undergo a C/S before 39 weeks.

Late Preterm (34 0/7–36 6/7)
- Placenta previa with suspected accreta, increta, or percreta
- Di–di twins with growth restriction and other maternal comorbidity
- Mo–di twins with growth restriction
- Preeclampsia—severe
- PPROM

Late Preterm (34 0/7–36 6/7) to Early Term (37 0/7–38 6/7)
- Placenta previa
- Prior classical cesarean
- Growth restriction with another complication such as oligohydramnios or a maternal comorbidity
- Di–di twins with growth restriction
- Mo–di twins
- Twins with oligohydramnios
- Chronic hypertension difficult or uncontrolled
- Diabetes pregestational/gestational uncontrolled

Early Term (37 0/7–38 6/7)

- Di–di twins
- Gestational hypertension
- Preeclampsia—mild

Early Term (37 0/7–38 6/7) to Term (39 0/7–40 6/7)

- Prior myomectomy
- Growth restriction
- Chronic hypertension—no medication needed or controlled on medication
- Pregestational with vascular complications
- Antibiotics—If PPROM
    - Ampicillin 2 g IV Q 6 hr × 48 hr, then
    - Erythromycin (Erythrocin) 250 mg IV Q 6 hr × 48 hr

Fast Facts

Antidote (hypermagnesemia): Calcium gluconate 1 g IV over 3 min; Rapid infusion can result in cardiac arrest. **Should be in room if MgSO4 is infusing.** RN does not need to be in the room for full infusion time.

Sources

Hurt, K. J., Guile, M. W., Bienstock, J. L., Fox, H. E., & Wallach, E. E. (2020). *The Johns Hopkins manual of gynecology and obstetrics* (6th ed.). Lippincott Williams & Wilkins.

Delnord, M., & Zeitlin, J. (2019). Epidemiology of late preterm and early term births: An international perspective. *Seminars in Fetal and Neonatal Medicine, 24*(1), 3–10. https://doi.org/10.1016/j.siny.2018.09.001

King, T. L., Brucker, M. C., Osborne, K., & Jevitt, C. M. (2019). *Varney's midwifery* (6th ed.). Jones & Bartlett Learning.

SHOULDER DYSTOCIA

- Obstetrical emergency
- The fetus's anterior shoulder is lodged behind the woman's pubic bone

Risk Factors

- Maternal hx of shoulder dystocia with previous deliveries
- Macrosomia
- Gestation diabetes and type 1 diabetes
- Maternal obesity
- Postdates
- Undiagnosed cephalopelvic disproportion (CPD)

Clinical Presentation

- Turtle sign is a classic sign of an impending shoulder dystocia (after the head emerges from the vagina, it quickly retracts)
- Dysfunctional second stage or active phase of labor (not always seen)
- Protracted labor (dilating less than 1 cm/hr)
- Failure to descend

Whom to Call

- GET HELP IMMEDIATELY
- Call covering physician STAT if midwife is managing patient
- Notify pediatrician STAT
- Notify anesthesia STAT
- Call all senior nursing staff available to help

Fast Facts

Always have a step stool in the delivery room. Call for a second RN to be in room for macrosomia precautions. Always watch family/support people in the room—they may be traumatized and pass out.

What to Do

- Instruct mother *not* to push until instructed to do so; explain there is a problem and provide reassurance
- Strategies that may serve to alleviate or dislodge shoulder dystocia
- McRoberts maneuver: bring the mother's legs all the way back in an exaggerated lithotomy position (this will open the diameter of the pelvis)

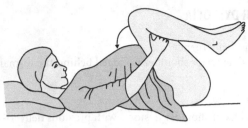

Lithotomy position

- Apply suprapubic pressure: ask the practitioner which way the back is; angle pressure diagonally against fetal back in attempt to collapse the anterior shoulder
  - Do not press straight down

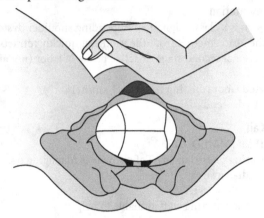

Suprapubic pressure

- Be prepared to readjust and do McRoberts maneuver again
- Gaskin position: hands and knee position may be requested by the practitioner; assist the mother into this position (if able, if not under heavy effects of epidural anesthesia)

Fast Fact

NEVER apply fundal pressure.

What the Physician and/or Midwife Is Doing
- Although the RN is aiding with the dislodgment of the shoulder externally, the practitioner is attempting to use internal maneuvers to dislodge the shoulders

- Rubin's maneuver: internally trying to collapse anterior shoulder to dislodge from pubic bone

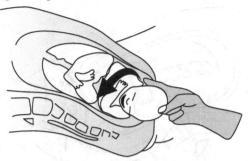

Rubin's maneuver

- Woods's screw maneuver: rotating the posterior shoulder into anterior position to facilitate delivery of the neonate

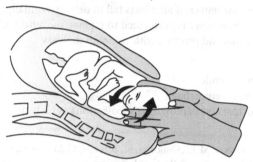

Woods's screw maneuver

- Reverse Woods's screw maneuver: similar to Woods's screw maneuver but rotating in opposite direction

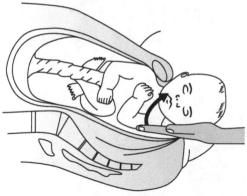

Reverse Woods's
screw maneuver

- Delivery of the posterior arm: sweeping the posterior arm across the fetal chest delivering the position the shoulder first

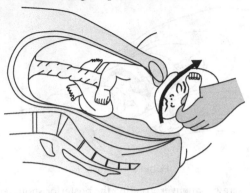

Delivery of the posterior arm

- Zananelli maneuver: if all efforts fail to deliver vaginally, the Zananelli maneuver is performed to replace the fetus back into the vaginal canal and proceed with cesarean delivery

Anticipate
- Full neonate code
- Postpartum hemorrhage
- Have postpartum hemorrhage medications at bedside

Sources
King, T. L., Brucker, M. C., Osborne, K., & Jevitt, C. M. (2019). *Varney's midwifery* (6th ed.). Jones & Bartlett Learning.

South Australian Perinatal Practice Guidelines. (2010). *Shoulder dystocia.* www.health.sa.gov.au/PPG/DEFAULT.aspx?PageContentMode=1&tabid=210

UMBILICAL CORD PROLAPSE

Fetal blood supply is compromised because the umbilical cord has slipped through the cervix ahead of the presenting part (frank) or has slipped alongside of presenting part (occult). Both are medical emergencies, and a STAT cesarean delivery should be anticipated.

Risk Factors
- Preterm
- Polyhydramnios
- Multiple gestations
- ROM before fetal head is engaged in pelvis
- Malpresentation

Clinical Presentation
- Usually occurs immediately after ROM
- Prolonged bradycardia
- Severe variable decelerations
- Umbilical cord palpable on vaginal exam
- Visualization of cord inside vagina
- Visualization of cord prolapsing from vagina

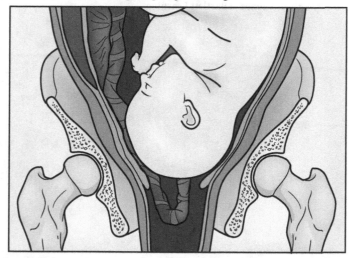

Cord Prolapse

Whom to Call
- GET HELP IMMEDIATELY
- Call the covering physician STAT if the midwife is managing the patient

- Notify the pediatrician STAT
- Notify anesthesia STAT
- Notify the OR staff

What to Do

- Occult cord: position mother in knee-to-chest or Trendelenburg position
- Continue to attempt to assess FHR either through EFM, ISE (if previously placed), or U/S
- Frank cord: place hand in vagina and push presenting part off the cord
  - DO NOT REMOVE HAND FROM VAGINA until instructed to do so by the practitioner during C/S
- Wrap cord in towel soaked with warm normal saline
- Anticipate STAT C/S

Sources

Hurt, K. J, Guile, M. W., Bienstock, J. L., Fox, H. E., & Wallach, E. E. (2020). *The Johns Hopkins manual of gynecology and obstetrics* (6th ed.). Lippincott Williams & Wilkins.

King, T. L., Brucker, M. C., Osborne, K., & Jevitt, C. M. (2019). *Varney's midwifery* (6th ed.). Jones & Bartlett Learning.

Appendix A

ABBREVIATIONS

ACOG	American College of Obstetricians and Gynecologists
AFI/AFV	amniotic fluid index/volume
AFP	alpha fetoprotein
AROM	artificial rupture of membranes
ASCUS	atypical squamous cells of undetermined significance
B-Hcg	beta-human chorionic gonadotropin
BID	two times a day
BP	blood pressure
bpm	beats per minute
BPP	biophysical profile
BV	bacterial vaginosis
c/o	complaint of
C/S	cesarean section
C&S	culture and sensitivity
CBC	complete blood count
CC	chief complaint
CF	cystic fibrosis
CIN	cervical intraepithelia neoplasia
CM	certified midwife
CMT	cervical motion tenderness
CMV	cytomegalovirus
CNM	certified nurse midwife
CNS	central nervous system
colpo	colposcopy
complete	10 cm dilated
CP	cerebral palsy
CPD	cephalopelvic disproportion

CT	*Chlamydia trachomatis*
ctx	uterine contractions
CVS	chorionic villa sampling
CXR	chest x-ray
d/c	discontinue
d/t	due to
D&C	dilatation and curettage
DES	diethylstilbestrol
DIC	disseminated intracoagulopathy
DKA	diabetic ketoacidosis
DM	diabetes mellitus
DOB	date of birth
DTR	deep tendon reflex
DVT	deep vein thrombosis
dx	diagnosis
EDC/EDD	estimated date of confinement/delivery date
EFM	electronic fetal monitoring
EFW	estimated fetal weight
F/U	follow-up
fFN	fetal fibronectin
FHR/FHT	fetal heart rate/tones
FKC	fetal kick count
FOB	father of baby
FSE	fetal scalp electrode
g	gram
GA	gestational diabetes
GBS	group B *Streptococcus*
GC	gonorrhea
GCT	glucose challenge test
GDM	gestational diabetes mellitus
GTT	glucose tolerance test
GU	genitourinary
GYN	gynecological
H/A	headache
Hb	hemoglobin
HCT	hematocrit
HDN	hemorrhagic disease of the newborn
HEENT	head, ears, eyes, nose, throat
h/o	history of
HPI	history of present illness
HPV	human papilloma virus
hs	hour of sleep
HSIL	high-grade squamous intraepithelial lesions
HSV	herpes simplex virus

HTN	hypertension
hx	history
IA	intermittent auscultation
IDDM	insulin-dependent diabetes mellitus
IM	intramuscular
IP	intrapartum
ISE	internal scalp electrode
ITP	idiopathic thrombocytopenia
IU	international units
IUFD	intrauterine fetal demise
IUGR	intrauterine growth restriction
IUI	intrauterine insemination
IUP	intrauterine pregnancy
IUPC	intrauterine pressure catheter
IV	intravenous
IVF	in vitro fertilization
IVPB	intravenous piggyback
L/S	lecithin/spinogomyelin
LBW	low birth weight
LGA	large for gestational age
LMP	last menstrual period
LSIL	low-grade squamous intraepithelial lesions
mcg	microgram
mg	milligram
mL	milliliter
MSAFP	maternal serum alpha fetoprotein
multip	multiparous
MVU	Montevideo units
N/V	nausea/vomiting
neg	negative
NPO	nothing by mouth
NSAID	nonsteroidal anti-inflammatory drug
NST	nonstress test
NSVD	normal spontaneous vaginal delivery
NT	nontender
NTD	neural tube defect
nullip	nulliparous
OTC	over the counter
PE	physical exam
PGE 1	prostaglandin
pgy 1, 2, etc.	resident postgraduate year 1, 2, 3, or 4
PIH	pregnancy-induced hypertension
pit	Pitocin
plt	platelet

PO	by mouth
POC	products of conception
pos	positive
PPD	purified protein derivative (test for TB)
PPH	postpartum hemorrhage
PPROM	preterm premature rupture of membranes
PR	by rectum
primip	primiparous
PRN	as needed
PROM	premature rupture of membranes
pt	patient
PTB/PTD	preterm birth/delivery
PTL	preterm labor
PV	per vagina
q	every
QD	one time per day
QHS	at hour of sleep
QID	four times per day
QOD	every other day
RDS	respiratory distress syndrome
RhoGAM	$Rh_o(D)$ immunoglobulin
r/o	rule out
ROM	rupture of membranes
ROS	review of systems
RR	respiratory rate
RRR	regular rate and rhythm
RTC/RTO	return to clinic/office
s/s	signs and symptoms
S>D	size greater than dates
S<D	size less than dates
SAB	spontaneous abortion
SOB	shortness of breath
SROM	spontaneous rupture of membranes
SSE	sterile speculum exam
STI	sexually transmitted infection
SVE	sterile vaginal exam
SX	surgery
TB	tuberculosis
TID	three times per day
TOC	test of cure
TPAL	T = term deliveries ≥37 weeks
	P = preterm deliveries <37 weeks
	A = abortion (elective or spontaneous) >20 weeks
	L = living children

TVU	transvaginal ultrasound
tx	treatment
U	units
UCX	uterine contractions
UPI	uterine placental insufficiency
U/S	ultrasound
UTI	urinary tract infection
VBAC	vaginal birth after cesarean section
VS	vital signs
WNL	within normal limits

Appendix B

AN ALPHABETIC SYNOPSIS OF MEDICATIONS COMMONLY USED IN PREGNANT AND POSTPARTUM WOMEN

Type of medication - generic (trade)	Indication	Contraindication	Dosage	Nursing implications
Betamethasone (Celestone Soluspan)	Risk for preterm birth; promotes fetal lung maturation	Allergy to drug	12 mg IM once daily × 2 d given 24 hr prior to birth if possible	Administer in gluteal muscle, assess blood pressure, edema, and weight. Monitor glucose levels and WBC if woman at risk for infection.
Carboprost tromethamine (Hemabate)	Reduces blood loss related to uterine atony	Acute cardiac, pulmonary, or renal disease	250 mg IM repeated every 1.5–3.5 hr. Total dose ≤12 mg in 24 hr; use should be limited to 48 hr	Monitor temperature, blood pressure, pulse, adverse side effects.
Dinoprostone (Cervidil)	Ripening of unfavorable cervix when delivery is indicated	Previous uterine surgery, sensitivity to prostaglandins, nonreassuring fetal status, bleeding of undetermined origin, suspected cephalopelvic disproportion, oxytocin infusion in use, contradictions for vaginal birth	Single vaginal insert containing 10 mg dinoprostone	Administer far back in posterior fornix of vagina, maintain bedrest for 2 hr after insertion, vaginal insert should be removed after 12 hr or if hypersystole or nonreassuring fetal status occurs, monitor vital signs, and ongoing cervical assessments to document progress.

Misoprostol (Cytotec)	Ripening of unfavorable cervix when delivery is indicated	Nonreassuring fetal status, previous uterine surgery, placenta previa, undiagnosed vaginal bleeding		Continuous fetal monitoring is warranted, oxytocin should not be started until at least 4 hr after last dose.
Dinoprostone (Preidil)	Cervical ripening and to promote uterine contractions when delivery is indicated	Nonreassuring fetal status, previous uterine surgery, unexplained vaginal bleeding, oxytocin infusion in place, multiparity >6, cephalopelvic disproportion, contraindications to vaginal birth	0.5 mg dinoprostone in 2.5 mL gel	Monitor contractions, vital signs, and cervical changes.
Magnesium sulfate	Used to treat neurological irritability, relax smooth muscle which decreases blood pressure, and decreases frequency and duration of uterine contractions	Myasthenia gravis is an absolute contraindication. Cautious use in heart block, heart damage, and impaired renal functioning	Loading dose is 4–6 g over 20–30 min, then 2–3 g/hr via infusion pump	Monitor blood pressure throughout administration, frequent vital signs, hourly urine output monitoring via Foley catheter, assess DTRs every hour, continuous fetal monitoring is warranted, magnesium levels every 6–8 hr to establish therapeutic range and monitor for toxic levels.

(continued)

AN ALPHABETIC SYNOPSIS OF MEDICATIONS COMMONLY USED IN PREGNANT AND POSTPARTUM WOMEN

Type of medication - generic (trade)	Indication	Contraindication	Dosage	Nursing implications
Methylergonovine maleate (Methergine)	Stimulates smooth muscle of uterus to sustain a contracted state of the uterus postpartum; decreases heavy bleeding related to uterine atony	Hypertensive disorders, use with caution with hepatic, liver, or cardiac diseases and sepsis	IM dose 0.2 mg–0.4 mg every 2–4 hr up to 5 doses, oral dose 0.2 mg–0.4 mg every 6–12 hr for 2–7 d	Monitor for side effects, vital signs, and bleeding. Administer pain medications to counter pain associated with uterine cramping. Advise women not to smoke during use of medication.
Nifedipine (Procardia)	A smooth muscle relaxer used for off-label use to reduce uterine contractions during preterm labor	Allergy to medication, hypotension, hepatic dysfunction, concurrent use of beta-mimetics or MgSO4, transdermal nitrates, or other antihypertensive medication	Initial dosage is 20 mg orally, followed by 20 mg orally after 30 min. If contractions persist, therapy can be continued with 20 mg orally every 3–8 hr for 48–72 hr with a maximum dose of 160 mg/d after 72 hr	Continuous fetal heart rate monitoring, contraction pattern, and maternal vital signs including pulse and blood pressure should be regularly monitored. Assess for side effects during administration.

Drug	Action	Contraindication	Dosage	Nursing considerations
Oxytocin (Pitocin) for postpartum administration	Stimulates uterine contractions during the third and fourth stage of labor to aid in the birth of the placenta and to control postpartum bleeding or hemorrhage	Hypersensitivity to the drug	Intramuscular dose is 1 mL (10 U) of Pitocin after the delivery of the placenta. Intravenous infusion is 10–40 U of oxytocin may be added to 1-L bottle of intravenous solution with the drip rate adjusted to a dose that sustains adequate uterine contractility and controls uterine atony	Continue to monitor for uterine atony, presence of clots, and heavy bleeding. Due to excessive cramping, pain medications may be administered. Women with a scar on their uterus should be monitored for symptoms of uterine rupture. Ongoing bleeding when the uterus is firm requires consultation to rule out other sources of bleeding such as sulcus tears or cervical laceration.
Terbutaline (Brethine)	A tocolytic used to stop premature contractions or tachysystole that occurs in connection with labor, typically related to Pitocin induction or augmentation	Sensitivity to the drug, heart disease, hyperthyroidism, and poorly controlled diabetes *See FDA Black Box Warning information	Dosage is 10 mg–40 mg with a maximum dosage of 40 mg per 24 hr. Subcutaneous dose 0.25 mg every 20–60 min until contractions have subsided is normal regimen	Continuous electronic fetal heart rate and contraction monitoring. Routinely assess lung sounds and vital signs. Assess for side effects and report immediately if they occur. Monitor length of treatment and notify provider if treatment regimen approaches 72 hr.

(continued)

AN ALPHABETIC SYNOPSIS OF MEDICATIONS COMMONLY USED IN PREGNANT AND POSTPARTUM WOMEN

Type of medication - generic (trade)	Indication	Contraindication	Dosage	Nursing implications
Ondansetron (Zofran)	Can be used to treat nausea and vomiting following birth	History of heart arrhythmias	4 mg every 4–6 hr PRN for nausea and vomiting	Women with severe nausea and vomiting warrant frequent weight monitoring, urine dips for ketones, and laboratory monitoring. Watch for severe dehydration and electrolyte imbalance.

*Black Box Warning: An FDA warning in 2011 noted that oral terbutaline should not be used for the treatment of preterm labor contractions and that the use of subcutaneous administration should be limited. Maternal death and serious adverse reactions, including tachycardia, transient hyperglycemia, hypokalemia, arrhythmias, pulmonary edema, and myocardial ischemia, have been reported, prompting the new guidelines. Recommendations for short-term use up to 48 to 72 hours to delay birth so corticosteroids can be administered is still supported although once contractions have been halted; long-term use of nifedipine or another tocolytic may be warranted.

Adapted from Davidson, M. R. (2014). *Fast facts for the antepartum and postpartum nurse.* Springer Publishing Company.

EMERGENCY DRUGS

Indication	Drug name—generic (trade)	Dosage, route, and frequency	Comments/cautions
Preterm labor			
Corticosteroids (for fetal lung maturity)			
	Betamethasone (Celestone)	12 mg IM q 12 hr × 2 doses	
	Dexamethasone	6 mg IM q 12 hr × 4 doses	
Tocolytics (to try to stop labor)			
	Indomethacin (Indocin)	50–100 mg PO at first dose, then 25–50 mg PO q 4–6 hr	Do not give if oligohydramnios
	Nifedipine (Procardia)	10–20 mg PO q 6 hr	
	Terbutaline	0.25 mg SQ q 20–30 min PRN	May cause maternal tachycardia
	Magnesium sulfate	Loading dose: 4–6 g IV, then 2–4 g IV/hr	Serum magnesium (Mg) level should be drawn q 6 hr
			Levels should be between 6 and 8 mg/dL
			Levels 8–10 mg/dL + decrease deep tendon reflexes
			Levels 13–15 mg/dL + respiratory distress
			Levels >15 mg/dL + cardiac arrest

(continued)

Indication	Drug name—generic (trade)	Dosage, route, and frequency	Comments/cautions
			Monitor I&O Manage IV drip so no more than 125 mL/hr infuses
			ANTIDOTE: calcium gluconate 1 g IV over 3 min
Postpartum haemorrhage			
	Oxytocin (Pitocin)	10 IU/mL IM or 40 U IV	Should have drug in room at every delivery
	Methylergonovine (Methergine)	0.2 mg IM q 2–4 hr	Do not give to hypertension (HTN)/preeclamptic patients
			Keep in refrigerator
	Carboprost (Hemabate)	250 mcg IM q 15–90 min; maximum 8 doses	Do not give to patients with history of asthma
	Misoprostel (Cytotec)	800–1,000 mcg rectal	
Preeclampsia			
	Magnesium sulfate	Loading dose: 4–6 g IV, then 2–4 g IV/hr	Serum magnesium (Mg) level should be drawn q 6 hr
			Levels should be between 6 and 8 mg/dL
			Levels 8–10 mg/dL + decrease deep tendon reflexes
			Levels 13–15 mg/dL + respiratory distress
			Levels >15 mg/dL + cardiac arrest
			Monitor I&O

Labetalol (Trandate)	20 mg IV push then increase dose at 10 min intervals to 20, 40, 80 mg, for max 30 mg/24 hr	Manage IV drip so no more than 125 mL/hr infuses
		ANTIDOTE: calcium gluconate 1 g IV over 3 min
Hydralazine	5 mg IV bolus q 20 min until 20 mg PRN	NOT FOR RN ADMINISTRATION

Opioid-addicted mother (for nonresponsive or low-Apgar neonate)

| Nalozone | 0.1 mg/kg IV, IM, or SQ, q 2–3 min PRN | Pediatrician should be at delivery |

Appendix C

GENERAL CHARTS

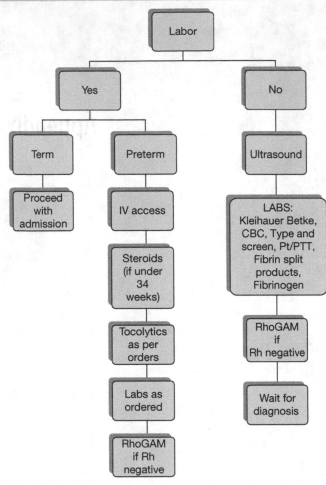

Bleeding in pregnancy

ANTEPARTUM TESTS

Initial Visit 8 to 12 Weeks

- U/S for dating
- Pap
- Blood type/Rh factor
- Antibody screen
- GC/CT
- Complete blood count (CBC)
- Syphilis
- HIV
- Hep B
- Rubella titer
- UA
- Hemoglobin electrophoresis
- Cystic fibrosis
- Varicella titers
- Toxoplasmosis
- Cytomegalovirus (CMV)
- Blood glucose (if overweight or history of GDM)

U/S, ultrasound; UA, urinalysis; GC/CT, gonorrhea/*Chlamydia trachomatis*; GDM, gestational diabetes mellitus.

11 to 13 Weeks
- First-trimester screening (blood work and U/S) for early detection of Down syndrome
- CVS if needed

15 to 18 Weeks
- AFP for early detection of neural tube defects
- QUAD if no first trimester screening done or if increased risk for Down syndrome
- Amniocentesis if needed (most commonly done between 16 and 22 weeks)
- Glucose screening if patient has high-risk factors, including obesity, hx of GDM, family hx

20 Weeks
- U/S for fetal anatomy

28 Weeks
- If patient is Rh negative, RhoGAM should be administered (repeat blood type and Rh factor before administration)
- CBC
- HIV in some states or in high-risk women
- Glucose test

34 to 36 Weeks

- GBS (test accurate only for 5 weeks if done at 34 weeks and delivering at 41 weeks; consult with the provider if they want to repeat test)
- GC/CT
- Syphilis
- NST/BPP for advanced maternal age, obesity, GDMA, HTN, and other maternal factors such as drug abuse

TREATMENT IN PRETERM LABOR

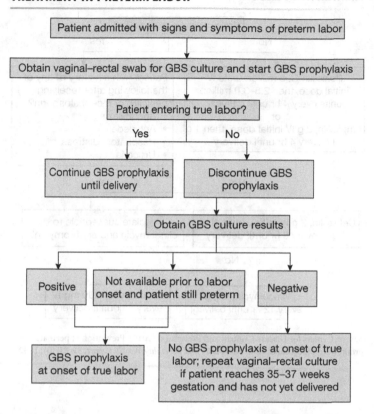

Source: Centers for Disease Control and Prevention (2010). Prevention of perinatal group B streptococcal disease. *Morbidity and Mortality Weekly Report*, *59*(RR10), 1–32.

If patient has PPROM, swab and treat for 48 hours.

TREATMENT IN LABOR

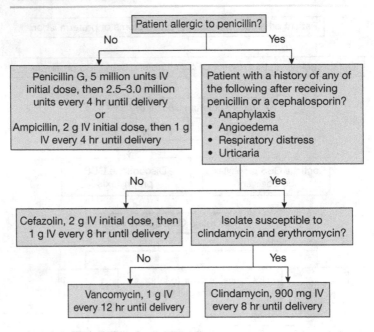

Source: Centers for Disease Control and Prevention (2010). Prevention of perinatal group B streptococcal disease. *Morbidity and Mortality Weekly Report, 59*(RR10), 1–32.

APGAR SCORE

- A score between 0 and 2 measuring heart rate, muscle tone, respiration rate, color, and reflex of the neonate at 1, 5, and 10 minutes of life

Breathing		
0	1	2
Not breathing	Slow irregular	Crying
Heart rate		
0	1	2
No heartbeat	Less than 100	Greater than 100
Muscle tone		
0	1	2
Floppy	Some tone	Active movement
Reflex/Grimace		
0	1	2
No response	Facial grimace only	Pulls away, cries, coughs, or sneezes
Skin color		
0	1	2
Pale blue	Body pink, hands and feet blue	Entire body is pink

SCORING THE APGAR

- 1 minute
    - Apgar scores are not indicative of future fetal well-being
- 5 minutes
    - 0 to 3 may indicate future neurological problems
    - 4 to 6 intermediate scores
    - 7 to 10 considered normal scoring range
- 10 minutes
    - Should continue to be assessed every 5 minutes if Apgar remains less than 7

BISHOP SCORE

Scoring system used to determine whether a cervix is inducible or which induction method would be most successful for a vaginal delivery.

	Bishop score			
Cervix	**0**	**1**	**2**	**3**
Dilation	0 cm	1–2 cm	3–4 cm	>5 cm
Effacement	0%–30%	40%–50%	60%–70%	80%
Station	−3	−2	−1/0	+1/+2
Consistency	Firm	Medium	Soft	
Position	Posterior	Mid	Anterior	

Index

Printed in the United States
by Baker & Taylor Publisher Services

Printed in the United States
by Baker & Taylor Publisher Services